TREATMENT OF
EDENTULOUS
PATIENTS

Commissioning Editor: Michael Parkinson
Project Development Manager: Clive Hewat
Project Manager: Frances Affleck
Designer: Erik Bigland

TREATMENT OF EDENTULOUS PATIENTS

J. Fraser McCord BDS DDS DRD FDS RCS(Ed) FDS RCS(Eng) CBiol MIBiol
Head of Department,
Unit of Prosthodontics, Turner Dental School, Manchester, UK

Phillip Smith BDS PhD DRD MRD FDS RCS(Ed) FDS (Rest Dent)
Lecturer/Consultant in Restorative Dentistry,
Unit of Prosthodontics, Turner Dental School, Manchester, UK

Nicholas Grey BDS MDSc PhD DRD MRD FDS RCS(Ed)
Consultant in Restorative Dentistry,
Unit of Prosthodontics, Edinburgh Dental Institute, Edinburgh, UK

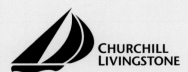

CHURCHILL LIVINGSTONE

EDINBURGH   LONDON   NEW YORK   OXFORD PHILADELPHIA   ST LOUIS   SYDNEY   TORONTO
2004

CHURCHILL LIVINGSTONE
An imprint of Elsevier Limited

First published 2004

ISBN 0443073074

British Library Cataloguing in Publication Data
A catalogue record for this book is available from the British Library

Library of Congress Cataloging in Publication Data
A catalog record for this book is available from the Library of Congress

Notice
Medical knowledge is constantly changing. Standard safety precautions must be followed, but as new research and clinical experience broaden our knowledge, changes in treatment and drug therapy may become necessary or appropriate. Readers are advised to check the most current product information provided by the manufacturer of each drug to be administered to verify the recommended dose, the method and duration of administration, and contraindications. It is the responsibility of the practitioner, relying on experience and knowledge of the patient, to determine dosages and the best treatment for each individual patient. Neither the Publisher nor the authors assume any liability for any injury and/or damage to persons or property arising from this publication.

The Publisher

ELSEVIER   your source for books,
journals and multimedia
in the health sciences
www.elsevierhealth.com

Printed in China

Preface

This textbook is intended to address the problems encountered by undergraduates and colleagues in those few years post graduation where the onus of clinical responsibility rests on the new clinician. Clinical demands are manifestly put to the test in the edentulous patient as these patients are subjected to dental, social and, often in the elderly, medical problems. The need to make a thorough assessment is of paramount importance as is the prerogative of measured decision – making and the prescription of appropriate treatment planning.

To assist the reader, we have attempted to formulate this textbook in such a way as to establish a sound template on how to formulate an appropriate treatment plan and, thereafter, to outline an overview of prosthodontic techniques which have been found to be of use by the authors.

To add to the educational value, Case Studies are included to illustrate how some basic prosthodontic techniques may be used to the advantage of the clinician, and, it is hoped, to promote a satisfactory outcome.

We live in an age where removable prosthodontic teaching occupies a significantly smaller percentage of teaching than previously. At the same time, the incidence of edentulousness is falling and the clinician has a need to be able to maintain the oral health of and to treat, with at least an aspiration of success, the edentulous patient.

We feel strongly that, in the case of edentulous patients particularly, it should be the domain of the dental surgeon to oversee the health of the remaining oral tissues, to maintain that health, to educate the patient on mouth care and, finally, to be able to provide treatment (or to refer appropriately) when replacement dentures are required. For that reason, the profession needs to be proficient in assessing the patient, determining which treatment option is important and also how to provide that treatment. The aim of this textbook is to help the reader to plan the treatment of edentulous mouths, in addition to explaining the prosthodontic principles behind some techniques.

Acknowledgements

A great deal of time and energy has gone into preparing this textbook which was prepared 'out of work hours' often into the wee small hours of the morning. Most clinicians will recognise the sacrifice that their families have had to make in order that fellowships, masters degrees or doctorates are 'bagged'. Further demands on family time are made when textbooks are undertaken and we wish to record our heartfelt appreciation to our wives, Morag, Kate and Sue for their unstinting encouragement. To all three plus our children, we apologise for our enforced absences and we dedicate this book to you all.

This textbook, in its present form, would not have occurred without the prompting, professionalism and perseverance of Janet Lear who had to deal with faulty typing, misspellings and different fonts. At the same time, she was encouraging and brimming with ideas on presentation. To Janet, we wish to express our deep gratitude.

We also wish to thank the following for their assistance:

Ray Richmond, Fraser Macauley and Patrick Brewer for their help with the technological aspects of some of the cases; Mike Parkinson and his team at Elsevier, and last, but by no means least, the many patients who contributed significantly to our clinical advancement.

This book is dedicated to Nick's dad, Terry.

Contents

1 Assessment of edentulous patients

The principal objective of prosthodontic treatment should be to satisfy each patient's functional and aesthetic requirements in the most effective and least traumatic way. In tandem with this, clinicians should also seek to establish and maintain each patient's mouth in a healthy state, as well as keeping any prosthesis/prostheses in a serviceable condition.

In addition to dental practitioners employing accepted clinical and technical standards in the production of prostheses, patient acceptance of complete dentures largely depends on their being able to make the necessary functional and psycho-social adaptations associated with successful denture wearing.

There is no guarantee that this ideal can be achieved in every case, but careful patient management demands that it should be at least addressed for all edentulous patients.

A crucial part of effective prosthodontic management revolves around being able to make a meaningful assessment of each patient in general, together with an assessment of his/her mouth and any current or previous prostheses specifically. This process then leads the dentist to determine whether patient expectations are reasonable and, therefore, likely to be met by current prosthodontic treatment strategies. On the other hand, it should also establish whether such expectations are unrealistic; some may not

be and as such are beyond what is currently achievable clinically. Such a process might hopefully prevent such patients from undergoing treatment where the prognosis is highly uncertain.

Prosthodontic assessment involves gathering information, not the analysis of this information, which then facilitates appropriate treatment planning in consultation with the patient and determining the likely prognosis for any proposed treatment.

INFORMATION GATHERING

Although this vital component of prosthodontic management should commence at first sight of the patient, it nevertheless depends upon the clinician taking a comprehensive history of the patient's presenting complaint together with detailed medical, dental and social histories. A physical inspection of the patient in general, a careful inspection and examination of the mouth and any dentures, plus any special investigations that might be appropriate in aiding a diagnosis, are also necessary. Although it is useful, in order to orientate the reader, to divide information gathering into discrete entities it is likely that experienced clinicians gather and analyse relevant information simultaneously. The important point is that all information relevant to patient management should be sought, considered and recorded. For simplicity, the remainder of this section will deal with information gathering and analysis together.

The presenting complaint and relevant history

This should be recorded, ideally, in the patient's own words, but the dentist should be careful to ensure that the meaning of the information being conveyed is clear. For example, the patient may complain about a denture being 'too big': this could mean that the denture is oversized, not a 'good fit' or, alternatively, that the artificial teeth appear too large to the patient.

The medical aphorism 'Let the patient speak: they will tell you the diagnosis' is pertinent. When patients are allowed to do this, the clinician will have a clearer picture of what their expectations are. It may also create a rapport between patient, clinician and the rest of the dental team. This is important in establishing a working partnership between patient and dentist, as this is one of the factors likely to determine whether a patient considers prosthodontic treatment to have been successful.

It is important that the dentist realises that attitude and behaviour have a marked influence on the consultation process. This means that the dentist needs to use appropriate body language and that a caring attitude is displayed towards the patient. Also of importance is **how** questions are phrased and used in order to allow the clinician to control and direct the consultation process. Thus although it is important to give patients adequate time, the interview ought to be structured in such a way as to allow the necessary information to be gathered in an efficient manner. Asking the patient whether they have any questions is a useful way to terminate the consultation, as it allows the patient to raise any concerns they may have, or alternatively to revisit any areas previously touched on.

Previous dental history

Reviewing the dental history provides much valuable information, not only about the oral condition but also about the patient's attitude to dental treatment. It is important not only for the dentist to determine when and why the natural teeth were lost, but also how the patient feels about the loss of his/her natural teeth.

Natural teeth lost through caries may indicate that they had acceptable bone support at the time of extraction and the residual ridges may be more favourable; conversely, teeth lost through periodontitis may lead the clinician to expect to see poorer (i.e. smaller) residual ridges. Whatever the reason for tooth loss, if a patient has undergone recent extractions the denture-bearing areas will still be remodelling, and this might therefore influence prosthodontic management.

Patients' feelings about their tooth loss should be sought in a compassionate manner, as many patients deeply regret this episode in their lives. For a minority, edentulousness is something that they find difficult to accept, and it comes to overshadow their ability to wear complete dentures successfully. Fortunately, most patients accept their edentulous state and are able to make the necessary functional and psychological adjustments in order to cope with complete dentures.

It is important to determine how patients have managed previous dentures when considering the provision of replacement prostheses. It is possible to envisage three prosthodontic scenarios:

- Previous dentures have been worn satisfactorily until problems developed recently.
- Initially dentures were successful, but more recent ones have been problematic.
- A history of several unsuccessful attempts at denture prescription.

Clearly the first two would appear to be easier to manage than the third, and it is important that patients realise from the start the limitations involved in wearing complete dentures and the not inconsiderable contribution they must make towards achieving a successful outcome to treatment. It is easy for unwary clinicians to embark on treatment that is unlikely to succeed unless an adequate assessment is made of previous denture-wearing history.

Health information

Health
1. Are you in good health?
2. Are you under the care of a doctor at the present time?
3. Have you ever had any serious illness or operation at any time?
4. Have you ever been in hospital, especially within the past year?

Illness
Do you suffer from, or have you had, any of the following:

Rheumatic fever?	Blackouts?
Rheumatic heart disease?	Fits?
Chorea (St Vitus dance)?	Fits or epilepsy?
Congenital heart disease (blue baby)?	Low blood pressure?
Heart murmur or valvular disease of the heart?	Asthma?
Anaemia?	Hay fever (summer colds)?
Heart trouble, heart attack?	Blocked nose
Stroke, paralysis or thrombosis?	Eczema or hives (urticaria)?
Tuberculosis?	Diabetes?
Bronchitis?	Jaundice (yellowing of the skin) especially after
Chest pains?	operation?
Persistent cough or shortness of breath?	Arthritis (rheumatism)?
Fainting spells?	Kidney trouble?

Medicines
1. Are you taking, or have you taken, any of the following medicines, tablets or drugs during the past year?
   (a) Antibiotics (penicillin, etc); (b) tablets for high blood pressure; (c) nerve tablets for depression; (d) insulin or others for diabetes; (e) anticoagulants (to thin the blood); (f) cortisone (steroids); (g) tranquillizers (sedatives); (h) digitalis etc. for the heart.
2. Do you habitually take alcohol?

Bad reactions
1. Are you, or have you been allergic, sensitive or hypersensitive to any drug, medicine or anything else, such as: (a) local anaesthetic; (b) penicillin or other antibiotic; (c) sleeping pills; (d) aspirin or similar pain-killing drugs; (e) sticking plaster; (f) iodine; (g) any other drug; (h) any type of food; (i) ointments.

Dental complications
1. Have you been treated by the dentist during the past 6 months?
2. Have you needed treatment for bleeding following dental extractions, operation or injury?
3. Do you bruise easily?
4. Are you employed in any situation which regularly exposes you to X-rays or other ionizing radiation?
5. Have you had any bad reactions to any form of dental treatment?
6. Have you or your relatives had any bad reactions to a general anaesthetic (going to sleep for an operation)?

For women
Are you pregnant or taking the contraceptive pill?

For patients of African or Mediterranean descent
1. Have you or members of your close family suffered with sickle cell anaemia or Cooley's anaemia?
2. Have you had a blood test for these diseases?

Fig. 1.1 Medical history pro-forma for patients.

Medical history

It is suggested that clinicians use a pro-forma (an example of which is given in Figure 1.1), which requires the patient to answer specific questions about her/his medical history. It might improve the level of information revealed if patients attended for consultation having completed this at home. This type of clinical approach ensures that all potentially important areas are covered, and the questionnaire then forms a useful starting point when patients are asked about their general health during the consultation appointment.

Apart from the influence systemic disease may have on dental management in general, illness may affect prosthodontic management either directly or indirectly, by influencing patient tolerance, adaptability or neuromuscular control. Clinicians are urged to consult with a patient's physician in all cases when systemic disease is thought likely to influence dental management. This might be the deciding factor as to whether treatment should proceed at all, or might require to be modified appropriately in order to take account of any health-related factors that may be present in any individual situation. It would be difficult to envisage a situation in which the provision of dental prostheses could justify damaging someone's general health; above all, the clinician must firstly 'cause no harm'.

Related to general health are those factors surrounding psychological health and motivation for dental treatment. It has been a long-held belief that psychological factors influence prosthodontic management.

House (1923) categorised prosthodontic patients into four personality types and suggested that personality greatly influenced whether a prosthesis was likely to be successful. Since this time, various studies have been conducted that have attempted to address this issue, which have reached conflicting conclusions (Fig. 1.2).

However, recent work has demonstrated that there is evidence to suggest that psychological factors and psychiatric illness have the potential to influence the outcome of prosthodontic treatment and certainly to affect patient management (Smith, 2001).

A minority of patients attend with dental and orofacial complaints for which there is no

Author	Personality Inventory	Summary
Watson & Reeve (1985) Reeve & Watson (1984)	Cattell 16PF	Showed relationship between personality and satisfaction with dentures
Watson et al (1986)	Cattell 16 PF	Similar results to above
Bolender et al (1969)	Cornell Medical index (CMI)	Increase in CMI score decreased denture satisfaction
Bolender et al (1969)	CMI	No relationship between CMI and post-insertion visits
Nairn & Brunello (1971)	CMI	Patients who complained more about their dentures scored higher in CMI
Guckes et al 1978	CMI	No correlation between CMI and satisfaction with dentures
Smith (1976)	Minnesota Multiphasic Personality Inventory (MMPI)	No correlation between satisfaction with denture and MMPI scores
Sobilik & Largon (1968)	MMPI	Showed relationship between MMPI scores and satisfaction with dentures
van Waas (1990)a	Health Locus of Control Scale (HCLS)	No relationship between HCLS and satisfaction with dentures
van Waas (1990)b	Wilde's Neurotic Liability Scale	Results similar to previous study

Fig. 1.2 Summary of studies using psychological inventories in prosthodontics.

apparent organic basis. An important part of patient assessment is to identify patients such as these who are unlikely to benefit from further dental intervention. Welsh et al. (2000) have shown the value of liaison psychiatry for a proportion of patients who suffer intolerance to dentures, and in some cases referral for psychiatric management could be an option. Patient acceptance of psychiatric intervention is of course variable, but uptake can be surprisingly high when appropriate referral mechanisms are in existence.

Social history

Social factors have the potential to influence the course and also the outcome of prosthodontic treatment. Patients usually attend alone for consultation, but often come with relatives or friends. The latter may lead clinicians to involve patients' relatives or friends in prosthodontic management, as this may provide valuable support for some patients. Conversely, other patients go to great pains to hide their true edentulous state and their wishes for 'prosthodontic privacy' should be respected. In addition, some patients often value the opinions of others who are close to them, particularly regarding their appearance. Their presence may be helpful for both clinician and patient, especially during the trial denture stage. Obviously there is a need to maintain confidentiality and to ensure that patients consent to this involvement.

Other aspects of the social history are also of importance, in particular the patient's ability to eat meals and the potential influence of dentures on the selection of particular foodstuffs. Patients may on occasion have unrealistic expectations about the type of food they expect to manage with their dentures: these patients will require careful counselling about the limitations of complete dentures before embarking on the construction of replacement prostheses.

Extraoral assessment

As was mentioned earlier, this begins on first seeing the patient. Often, subconsciously, the patient is assessed not only for her/his general condition but also her/his appearance in dentofacial terms, particularly in relation to the adequacy of vertical dimension and support for the facial tissues. It is at this stage that initial impressions are made of the likely tolerance of treatment and also regarding certain social factors that may be operating, such as the need to attend with relatives or carers. Dentists should be alert to any factors that might have a bearing on prosthodontic treatment:

- Frailty, which may influence patient tolerance of any planned changes in the prostheses, and the ability to attend for a series of appointments.
- Lack of mobility, which may mean the patient needs help to get into or out of the dental chair.
- Any obvious deficiency in hearing or sight that may require the use of communication aids.
- Obvious signs of dental or skeletal malrelationships that might influence the positioning of teeth or stability of dentures, for example marked Skeletal Class 2 or 3 jaw relationships (Figs 1.3, 1.4).
- Inappropriate facial vertical dimension may lead the clinician to expect the clinical sequelae related to overclosure, or alternatively a lack of freeway space (Fig. 1.5).
- In older patients who are spectacle wearers, an estimate of overall tissue tone may be

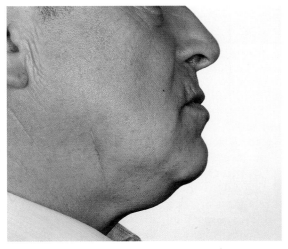

Fig. 1.3 This patient has a typical Class 3 profile.

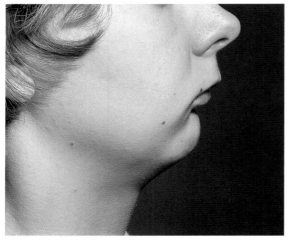

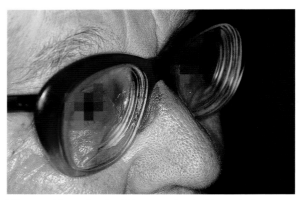

Fig. 1.6 Note the bruising on the bridge of the nose, suggestive of tissue fragility.

Fig. 1.4 This patient exhibits a typical Class 2 (division I) profile.

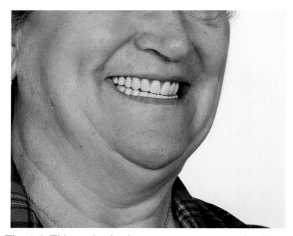

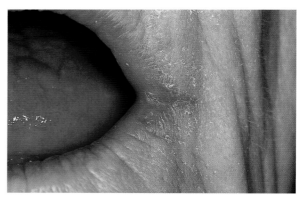

Fig. 1.7 Marked angular cheilitis. Note also the colour of the tongue.

Fig. 1.5 This patient's dentures were presented with an excessive occlusal vertical dimension.

gained from observation of tissues supporting spectacles (Fig. 1.6).

- The presence of angular cheilitis may alert the clinician to the presence of denture-induced stomatitis or systemic disease such as anaemia, poorly controlled diabetes or dietary deficiencies (Fig. 1.7). More likely is the presence of poorly fitting dentures coupled with poor oral and denture hygiene.

- The masticatory system should be assessed to see whether a normal range of pain-free excursive movements of the mandible is possible. The skin over the temporomandibular joints should be palpated and, if indicated, auscultation of the joints by means of a stethoscope to listen for joint sounds characteristic of temporomandibular disorders (Fig. 1.8). These may range from symptomless clicking to the characteristic crepitation of joints affected by osteoarthrosis.

- Careful observation of the patient while they are speaking will also yield valuable information that might influence prosthodontic management. Initial impressions regarding

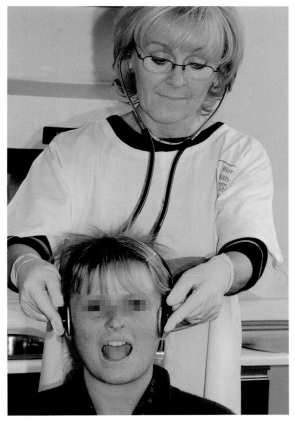

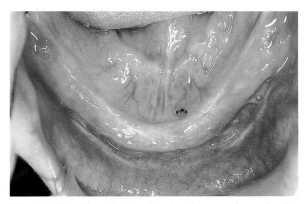

Fig. 1.9 The ridges, denture-bearing tissues and non-dentine tissues need to be assessed.

Fig. 1.8 Stereo stethoscope being used to listen for sounds in the temporomandibular joints.

Clinicians should routinely perform a full mouth examination in order to ensure that clinically detectable pathology is not overlooked. In particular, dentists should refer patients to the consultant in oral medicine or oral maxillofacial surgery if any suspicious or potentially malignant lesions are detected.

Denture-induced stomatitis is a relatively common finding in edentulous patients who wear ill-fitting prostheses. It is characterised by erythema of the denture-bearing area, and also may be accompanied by varying degrees of papillary hyperplasia (Fig. 1.10). It is important that this condition is recognised and appropriately managed prior to the provision of new dentures.

mandibular movement, and also tooth position in relation to phonetics, can be gained. For example, patients may exhibit marked forward translation of the mandible when speaking, and this should be taken into account by ensuring that the occlusion is balanced in mandibular protrusion, thereby reducing the potential for denture displacement.

Intraoral assessment

This should focus on whether the mouth is healthy, and also the likelihood of the remaining tissue adequately supporting, retaining and stabilising appropriately designed and adequately constructed prostheses (Fig. 1.9).

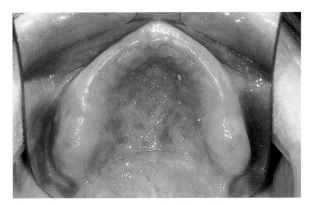

Fig. 1.10 Mild papillary hyperplasia is evident.

Once a careful general examination of the mouth has been undertaken, attention may then be transferred towards evaluating any potential denture-bearing areas. Despite many attempts to relate denture-bearing anatomy to patient satisfaction with dentures, it would appear that a clear relationship between the two is lacking (Slaghter 1992, van Waas 1990). By extrapolation, the dentist should not necessarily assume that what appears to be a plentiful ridge is a 'good ridge'.

However, despite the lack of a clear relationship between oral anatomical features and successful denture wearing, clinical experience suggests that specific strategies aimed at managing potential problems with support or retention appear to meet with some success.

The combination of well fitting and well functioning dentures, the absence of pain and a socially acceptable appearance contributes much to patients' satisfaction with complete dentures. Clearly, it is only possible to institute the appropriate clinical and technical strategies once the prevailing intraoral situation has been identified and assessed. Therefore, it is important that a careful inspection and palpation of the denture-bearing tissues is undertaken, aimed at eliciting any factors that might influence the support, retention or stability of the prosthesis/prostheses.

Factors to be borne in mind are as follows:

- The quantity and quality of saliva may be important for both patient comfort and denture retention. The lubricating nature of saliva may minimise the presence of microabrasions in the denture-bearing mucosa and act to improve patient comfort. The quality of saliva may influence the retention of dentures, especially the maxillary, by contributing to the forces of adhesion. Clinicians should be alert to the influence that systemic disease and various drugs may have on the production of saliva (Fig. 1.11).
- Retained roots or partially buried teeth which might require further attention and possibly removal (Fig. 1.12).
- Bony lumps and prominences which may require relief of the master casts (Fig. 1.13).

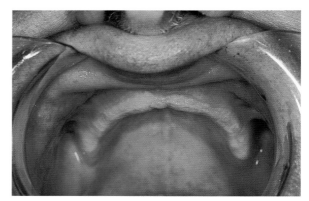

Fig. 1.11 This patient has a drug-induced dry mouth.

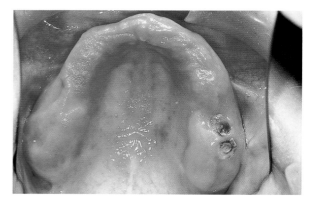

Fig. 1.12 The clinician must decide on the status of retained roots prior to commencing treatment.

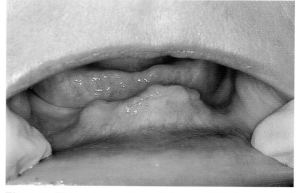

Fig. 1.13 This anterior ridge of the mandible has areas of undercut and also areas that will require relief.

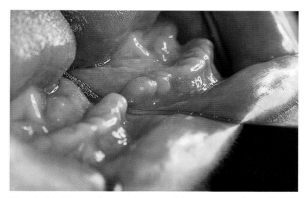

Fig. 1.14 This undercut ridge would indicate a planned path of insertion parallel to the ridge.

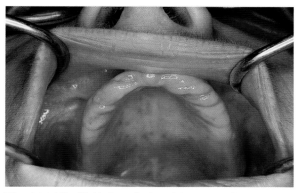

Fig. 1.16 The 'flabby' or displaceable nature of the anterior portion of the maxilla is evident.

- Undercuts which may dictate denture extension or the path of insertion (Fig. 1.14).
- Areas of the mouth which are tender to palpation and which may require relief of the denture bases, e.g. superficial inferior dental nerves in the region of the mental foramina (Fig. 1.15).
- Displaceable tissue, e.g. fibrous ridges, which may require the use of appropriate selective pressure impression techniques (Fig. 1.16).
- Enlarged tuberosities, which may indicate the need for elastic impression materials, or in a minority of cases surgical reduction (Fig. 1.17).
- Frenal or sulcular attachments close to the crest of the edentulous ridge which may interfere with peripheral extension (Fig. 1.18).

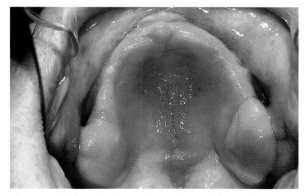

Fig. 1.17 Enlarged tuberosities reflect problems of planning for retention and stability.

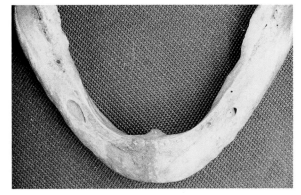

Fig. 1.15 The right mental foramen is particularly evident on this dried mandible. In patients with this degree of resorption, relief on the master cast is indicated.

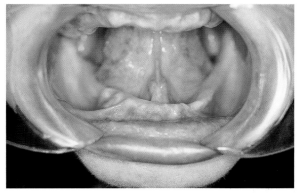

Fig. 1.18 The high muscle attachment on the (patient's) right would severely impair denture wearing.

As well as all of the above findings the clinician may also record the form of the mandibular and maxillary ridges. A good guide is that described by Attwood (1971).

- Class I corresponds to a good ridge prior to the extraction of teeth.
- Class II is the immediate post-extraction form of all the ridge.
- Class III is a well-rounded ridge form.
- Class IV is a knife-edged ridge.
- Class V is a flat ridge.
- Class VI is one where the resorption is such that there is a negative or concave form to the ridge surface.

The clinician should now be in a position to form an impression of the denture-bearing tissues and the form and nature of the associated peri-denture tissues in an attempt to assess the three fundamental features related to the provision of dentures. These are:

- Support
- Retention
- Stability.

According to Jacobson and Kroll (1983), they may be defined as:

- **Support**: That aspect of the denture-bearing tissues which resists displacement of the denture towards these tissues.
- **Retention**: That property of the denture-bearing and peridenture tissues that resists displacement of the denture away from these tissues.
- **Stability**: The property of the ridges per-dental musculature and the occlusal form of the dentures, which resists displacement of the denture at right-angles to the ridge (non-vertically).

Assessment of dentures

This should take into account the findings of the assessment so far. Although, historically, clinicians have attempted to assess the adequacy of various denture features, as yet no universally accepted index of denture needs has been developed (Pinsent & Laird 1989). This may be related to

the fact that prosthodontics is not an exact science but rather a blend of clinical skill and artistic flair (McCord & Grant 2000). To date, research has failed to demonstrate conclusively that denture quality affects patient satisfaction and hence denture success. However, there remains support for the important contribution that clinical–technical factors make towards successful treatment outcomes with complete dentures (van Waas 1990, Beck et al. 1993).

It would appear, therefore, that there are good reasons for existing and previous dentures to be carefully inspected both in situ and outside the mouth. The following aspects should be evaluated, as they may have an important bearing on patient management:

Inside the mouth

- Peripheral extension in relation to anatomical landmarks such as sulcus form, hard/soft palate junction, retromolar pads, retromylohyoid fossae. This requires careful observation of the denture while gently manipulating the lips and cheeks. Note should be made as to whether the denture is displaced while these movements are being performed, as this indicates over-extension and/or intrusion on muscle attachments. Equally important is to determine whether the denture peripheries are short of the sulcular reflection, thus indicating underextension (Fig. 1.19).

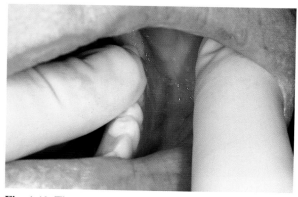

Fig. 1.19 The peripheries of each denture should be inspected to determine how they relate to the reflection of the sulcus.

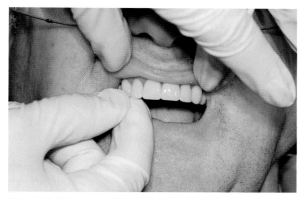

Fig. 1.20 Recommended method to determine retention of a denture.

- Retention of the upper denture may be empirically assessed by grasping the maxillary canines between fingers and thumb and attempting to rotate the denture out of the mouth (Fig. 1.20). A somewhat crude indication as to whether the denture resists this movement is gained; naturally, as the clinician gains experience in making this assessment the more reliable the judgement becomes. The retentive capacity of the lower denture is usually low, although it is possible to assess this by placing a probe into the embrasure between the central incisors and attempting to lift the lower denture vertically (Fig. 1.21).

- Stability may be gauged by attempting to depress the denture towards the denture-bearing tissues. This is readily achieved by placing finger pressure alternately on the occlusal surfaces of either side of the denture and observing whether it rocks or appears stable (Fig. 1.22). This could be related to the state of the supporting tissues, the impression technique employed, or deficiencies that might be present in the fitting surface of the dentures.

- Positioning of the artificial teeth in relation to the levels and orientation of occlusal planes, incisal level, angulation of the incisal plane and tooth arrangement. These factors not only have functional implications in terms of chewing comfort and denture stability, but also contribute to the overall appearance of dentures. Generally, the pattern of residual ridge resorption in the maxilla dictates that, in order to restore support for the facial tissues, the artificial teeth should be set labial to the ridge (Fig. 1.23). It is therefore important to take notice of the positioning of the teeth in relation to this, although the obvious exception is immediate complete dentures. Conversely, in order to enhance mandibular denture stability it is generally held that the central fossae of the lower posterior teeth, along with the necks of the mandibular anterior teeth, should lie over the crest of the residual mandibular ridge.

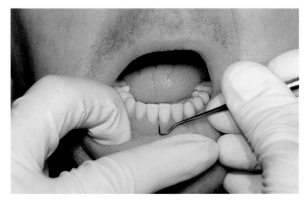

Fig. 1.21 Simple means of demonstrating the retentive capacity of a mandibular denture. NB: The patient should be instructed to keep her/his tongue flat here.

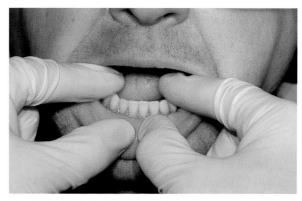

Fig. 1.22 Method of demonstrating one aspect of stability of this mandibular denture.

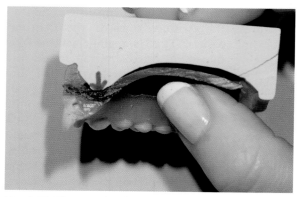

Fig. 1.23 The arrowhead marks the position of the midpoint of the incisive papilla. The compensation for loss of labial bone is apparent.

- Occlusal relationships also require assessment, as they have a bearing on denture stability, patient comfort and appearance. Initial assessment should be made as to whether simultaneous bilateral occlusal contact is made in the retruded jaw relationship. In some patients this may be facilitated by having the patient curl their tongue so the tip touches the posterior border of the maxillary denture, while at the same time elevating their mandible. It is important to see the first point of occlusal contact lest the mandible subsequently slides into a position in which there are more interocclusal contacts (Fig. 1.24). It is important to note whether such a slide occurs, as this may contribute to instability, especially of the lower denture. It is also helpful to assess whether smooth articulatory movements are also possible without causing the dentures to be displaced. Although many patients manage to chew with dentures that do not exhibit balanced articulation, for a minority this may be a requirement for successful denture wearing.

- Clinical experience suggests that the provision of an appropriate amount of freeway space is needed in order for patients to function comfortably with dentures (Fenlon et al. 1999). Not only does this parameter influence chewing and patient comfort, it also influences speech and appearance. It is determined by measuring the difference between the resting face height and the height of the face when the patient occludes in maximum intercuspation. However, it should be appreciated that owing to inconsistencies in the resting jaw position and the difficulties that may be encountered measuring facial height, the freeway space remains a useful estimate rather than an absolute value.

Outside the mouth

- Denture hygiene should be assessed by visual inspection and, if necessary, indicated by disclosing any plaque deposits (Fig. 1.25). Poor cleaning may relate to the development of denture-induced stomatitis or malodour, and

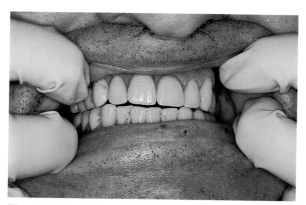

Fig. 1.24 There is an obvious premature contact on the patient's right side in RCP.

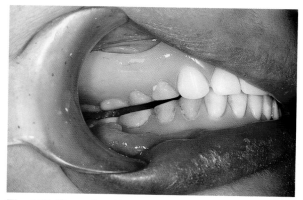

Fig. 1.25 Plaque is evident at the junction of the teeth with the denture base.

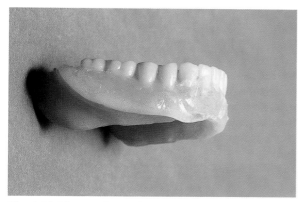

Fig. 1.26 Many patients who have resilient linings prefer to have them on their replacement dentures. This denture has a resilient lining.

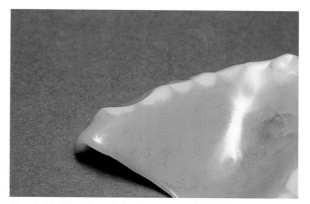

Fig. 1.27 The view of the denture teeth is indicative of parafunctional activity, especially as the dentures are over 2.5 years old. Subtle questioning is required to determine the nature of the habit.

all patients should receive advice regarding how best to maintain and clean their dentures.

- Materials used in denture construction should be considered, as these may indicate patient preferences, for example porcelain teeth, or support problems that have in the past necessitated the use of resilient denture base materials (Fig. 1.26).
- Signs of wear of the artificial teeth and bases may indicate dietary habits, such as the intake of confections containing peppermint oil, and parafunctional habits such as bruxism or pipe smoking, which may need to be taken into account when replacement dentures are being considered (Fig. 1.27).
- Impression surfaces should be carefully examined for any signs of relief included in the bases (Fig. 1.28), as these may indicate previous problems that have been encountered with supporting tissues.
- Tooth size, shape, colour and arrangement should be taken into account, particularly in the light of any comments the patient may make in relation to these.

More specific investigations

Classically these relate to radiological, haematological and microbiological investigations. In addition, certain prostheses could be viewed as diagnostic appliances, in that they may be used

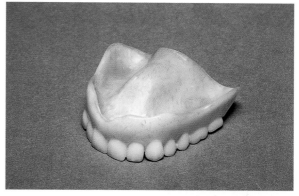

Fig. 1.28 The impression surface of this maxillary denture has been 'relieved' by the patient, as the dental team had not done so.

to assess patient tolerance and/or adaptation to changes in tooth position or occlusion. One example of this type of appliance is the 'pivot denture', which is used to determine stable jaw relationships that would be difficult to achieve via conventional jaw registration. The pivots are pillars of acrylic resin placed in the lower second premolar and first molar regions (see Case Study 2) and which are adjusted to allow contact with the palatal cusps of the upper premolar/molar teeth. This type of diagnostic appliance is especially useful in patients who have experienced difficulty in adapting to lower complete dentures, or who have difficulty reproducing consistent jaw relationships.

It is recognised that the mouth can be affected by a number of infections or manifestations of systemic disease, and that these may warrant further investigation and referral to a consultant in oral medicine as appropriate. However, as these lie outside the scope of this book the interested reader is referred to other texts that deal with these aspects more fully.

One of the conditions commonly encountered by the prosthodontist is that of denture-induced stomatitis related to candidal infection. This is usually effectively managed by a combination of denture hygiene, improved fitting of poorly adapted dentures, and the prescription of topical antifungal medication. On occasion it may be necessary to conduct haematological and micro-biological investigations, especially when protracted cases resist the usual therapeutic regimen. In these cases it is better to involve either a consultant in oral medicine, or alternatively the patient's general practitioner, in any further management, in case there are any underlying systemic factors that may have gone undetected.

Radiological investigations are not routinely indicated for patients who are completely edentulous. This follows the principle of good radiological practice in which radiographic investigation is required as a specific aid to diagnosis or treatment provision (National Radiographic Protection Board 2001). Examples would be the use of periapical radiographs to assess retained roots, or perhaps more sophisticated imaging such as computed tomography (CT) when planning the use of dental implants.

CONCLUDING REMARKS

As with any clinical discipline, treatment should only proceed once a thorough assessment and analysis of the clinical situation has been made. This should aim to elicit those factors that are thought to contribute to successful complete dentures (Fig. 1.29). Only then can the patient be advised of their choices and give their informed consent to what follows.

Equally, should a clinician be unsure about whether the expectations of the patient can be met, the appropriate course of action would be to withdraw from treatment and refer the patient to someone more appropriate.

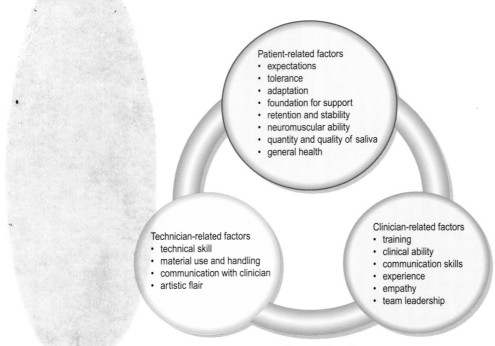

Patient-related factors
- expectations
- tolerance
- adaptation
- foundation for support
- retention and stability
- neuromuscular ability
- quantity and quality of saliva
- general health

Technician-related factors
- technical skill
- material use and handling
- communication with clinician
- artistic flair

Clinician-related factors
- training
- clinical ability
- communication skills
- experience
- empathy
- team leadership

Fig. 1.29 Summary of the factors contributing to successful complete dentures.

REFERENCES

Attwood DA. The reduction of residual ridges: a major oral disease entity. J Prosthet Dent 1971; 26: 266–270

Beck CB, Bates JF, Basker RM, Gutteridge DL, Harrison A. A survey of the dissatisfied denture patient. Eur J Prosthodont Rest Dent 1993; 2: 73–78

Fenlon MR, Sherriff M, Walter JD. Comparison of patients' appreciation of 500 complete dentures and clinical assessment of quality. Eur J Prosthodont Rest Dent 1999; 7: 11–14

House MM. An outline for examination of mouth conditions. Dom Dent J 1921; 33:97–100

Jacobson TE, Kroll AJ. A contemporary review of the factors involved in complete denture retention, stability and support. J Prosthet Dent 1983; 49: 5–15; 165–172; 206–313

McCord JF, Grant AA. A clinical guide to complete denture prosthetics. London: BDJ Books, 2000

National Radiographic Protection Board. Guidance notes for dental practitioners on the safe use of X-ray equipment. London: Department of Health, 2001

Pinsent RH, Laird WRE. Problems in the assessment of complete dentures. Commun Dent Health 1989; 6: 3–9

Slaghter AP. Masticatory ability, denture quality, and oral conditions in edentulous subjects. J Prosthet Dent 1992; 68: 299–307

Smith PW. Psychological aspects of complete denture wearing. PhD Thesis, University of Manchester, 2001

van Waas MAJ. The influence of clinical variables on patients' satisfaction with complete dentures. J Prosthet Dent 1990; 63: 307–310

Welsh G, Grey NJA, Potts S. The use of liaison psychiatry service in restorative dentistry. CPD Dentistry 2000; 1: 32–34

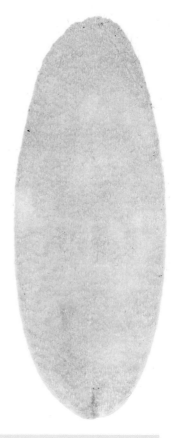

2 Decision-making and treatment options for the edentulous patient

As with any area of medicine and dentistry, the adage 'no diagnosis, no treatment' holds true for the edentulous patient. This statement has much validity in the management and treatment of edentulous patients. Although for the edentulous patient any error at the decision-making stage is unlikely to be fatal, the consequences of over-hasty or inaccurate decision-making/treatment planning may result in a less than ideal outcome. Corrective treatment post insertion may not resolve matters, as at that stage confidence may have been dissolved and a complaints procedure instigated.

The factors that determine decision-making for the edentulous patient are diverse. For example, many dentists will have experienced instances where two patients may have presented with two quite similar clinical scenarios yet two different treatment options will have been pursued. In an ideal world, should the two patients ever meet and ask for clarification from the dentist as to why their treatments differed, it ought to be possible for her/him to give a reasoned answer that withstands close scrutiny. Unfortunately, however, this is sometimes difficult, as the clinician may have made a decision based on 'clinical experience'. In the current climate of evidence-based dentistry, the validity of 'clinical experience' alone is being increasingly questioned.

The purpose of this chapter is to assist the reader in the decision-making process by outlining a series of possible treatment strategies, such that the treatment option selected for the patient is in fact the most appropriate for that patient.

Chapter 1 dealt with the assessment of the edentulous patient with respect to information gathering. When all the information has been assimilated, the dentist then has the task of using that information to arrive at a strategy that will best enable an optimal outcome. This must include a decision on what the aims of treatment are, and discussing these in depth with the patient.

There is no doubt that patients differ widely in what they want from dental treatment and this must be ascertained from the outset. There is no agreed definition of what exactly 'appropriate dentures' are, but we feel that this is best considered as 'a situation where the patient, after informed consultation with a dentist on all treatment options, makes a decision on her/his preferred treatment option – if this is feasible and within the competence of the clinician'.

In the general dental services of the National Health Service (United Kingdom), the nature of

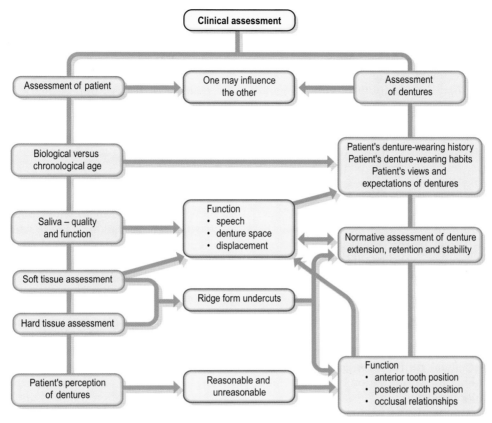

Fig. 2.1 A template that may be used to outline possible treatment scenarios.

remuneration rewards the dental practitioner only if treatment is carried out. Furthermore, the abilities of clinicians are often assessed by examination of cases of treated patients where treatment has actually been undertaken. This tends to endorse the fact that a satisfactory outcome may only be achieved by active intervention, and omits the fact that, on occasion, the option of no or minimal treatment may offer the best outcome.

A template for the various treatment options is illustrated in Figure 2.1 and it is suggested that the patient is encouraged to be part of the process of decision-making.

FACTORS INFLUENCING DECISIONS

There are many issues to consider that may affect the planning process.

Patient-related factors

A number of factors need to be addressed, and one of the first relates to the patient's reason for seeking treatment. McCord et al. (2002) considered some of the following reasons.

Appearance

Aesthetic problems that the patient perceives with present dentures may lead them to seek replacements, irrespective of 'fit' or comfort. Such problems may relate to the size, shape and colour of the teeth and are readily solved. However, problems relating to the position of the teeth may be more difficult to solve if the patient wishes the teeth to be placed in a position that could result in instability of the resultant denture. Typically, this occurs where unwanted age-related 'wrinkling' causes the patient to seek increased facial support.

In the case of the conventional complete mandibular denture, the placement of the anterior teeth/denture flange in a more anterior position than is physiologically desirable in order to fill out the face may result in denture instability, as the teeth/denture may be in conflict with the oral musculature. In such cases, reversible (diagnostic) treatment, such as the addition of wax to the existing denture to achieve the desired result, may allow an assessment to be made of the effect of such changes on the stability of the denture. If stability is likely to be compromised, the nature of the instability may be readily demonstrated to, and experienced by, the patient in a reversible way.

Patients may also feel that treatment is indicated because their denture/s look old or worn. If after careful assessment every other aspect of the dentures is perceived to be clinically satisfactory, replacement for this reason alone may result in future problems. Often, the dentures may be considered to have 'worn in' rather than to have been 'worn out'. In such cases, consideration should be given to the potential provision of replica (or template) dentures rather than replacements, to enable the continuation of the patient's neuromuscular control.

In the opinion of the authors, the dentist should be wary of injudicious prescription of relining and/or rebasing procedures for the established complete denture wearer, as the changes are irreversible. Although rare, the situation after a reline may sometimes be worse than before, and it is then virtually impossible to go back to square one. In such situations the patient may, quite rightly, blame the dentist, and to avoid this scenario it is recommended that use of a replica technique offers greater security, in that the patient may still be able to resort to their current dentures if the outcome of the relining of the replicas is not successful. Relining procedures are perhaps best considered for patients who have recently been supplied with immediate complete dentures, where postextraction residual ridge reduction may result in a poorer fit.

Function

It is understandable (although perhaps unrealistic) that denture wearers would wish to be able to function as well as they once did with their natural dentition. The patient may be asked how well they feel they should be able to function with their dentures. The response may allow an assessment to be made of whether her/his expectations are realistic. If they're not, then the dentist may elect not to proceed with treatment and offer an explanation as to why. An analogy may be made in that denture wearing is a little like skiing, the success being reliant on adequate neuromuscular control.

It is worth emphasising that the functional needs of the patient include eating, speech and swallowing, in addition to other habits, hobbies or pastimes, e.g. singing. These should all be considered when assessing the balance between what is expected and what possible.

Comfort

Given the inevitable and inexorable consequences of residual ridge resorption following the extraction of teeth, it is hardly surprising that discomfort is often reported by patients, especially in the mandibular arch, where the denture-bearing tissues are often minimal and atrophic in nature. Manual palpation may reveal areas where the tissue is not able to offer adequate support for a denture, such as atrophic mucosa, or flabby or knife-edge ridges. Management of such situations using specific impression techniques is outlined in Chapter 3, although the possibility of a resilient lining should be considered. Should such findings become evident during the examination stage, they should be mentioned to the patient as being significant in that they may make a satisfactory outcome more difficult to achieve. Although resilient linings often offer an immediate solution to the problem, the currently available materials do come with some disadvantages, in that their longevity is compromised. Resilient linings may be recommended when the patient insists on their use, usually after they have worn such linings previously.

Speech

Speech problems with complete dentures would not appear to be a large-scale problem but, for the few that are, such problems are difficult to manage. It is not the intention of this book to cover the management of speech difficulties in depth, but they generally arise from the setting of teeth in positions to which the patient cannot accommodate, or as a result of the morphology of the polished surfaces that causes interference with tongue movement.

For further information on speech problems, readers are referred to Grant et al. (1994).

Psychological

The next issue to be considered is that of the expectations of the patient. These may be ascertained by asking the patient simple questions and then listening carefully to what the patient wants. This may immediately reveal unrealistic expectations. Appelbaum, in 1984, commented: 'A patient with a false eye cannot see, a patient with false legs cannot run, yet a man with no teeth expects to be able to function with his dentures in much the same way as with his natural teeth'.

Where it becomes obvious to the dentist that the patient's expectations would not be addressed by active treatment it is better to explain this to the patient and refuse treatment, rather than embark on treatment with a strong likelihood of failure. This is often a very difficult decision to make, as it might suggest to the patient an inability rather than a reluctance on the part of the dentist to solve the problem. Although this may not be the case, it is better to address the situation and offer a balanced clinical decision at that stage than to have wasted the time, effort and cost of failed treatment.

Clinical factors

Many clinical factors may influence the outcome of treatment, including:

- The experience and ability of the dentist
- The experience and ability of the dental technician
- The presenting clinical features of the patient.

Chapter 1 deals with the clinical factors in more detail.

TREATMENT OPTIONS

In order to satisfy the medicolegal aspects of treatment, informed consent must be obtained before commencing. By extrapolation, therefore, it is essential that all treatment options be discussed with the patient to enable him/her to make an informed decision.

When all the above factors have been considered with all the information available, the plan can proceed and Anusavice (1992) reported that for good decision-making the clinician should:

- Reflect on the alternatives
- Become aware of the uncertainties
- Be able to modify his/her judgement on the basis of accumulated evidence
- Balance the judgement of the risks of various kinds
- Consider the possible consequences of each treatment option
- Synthesise all of the above factors in making a treatment decision.

With all of these factors in mind, the clinician has the following options either for patients fast approaching the edentulous state or for those who are already edentulous.

No treatment

As was discussed earlier, the decision not to provide treatment is a difficult one to take as it may be considered by the patient to imply a lack of ability on the part of the dentist – even if this is eminently not the case. The decision not to provide treatment should be made where the dentist considers that a result cannot be achieved that would satisfy the patient's expectations. This decision can only be made where the clinician has made a careful assessment of all clinical and perceptional factors pertinent to each patient, balanced with the combined skills of the dental team in its entirety.

It is important that the patient understands the reason/s for not providing treatment, and although he/she might not be content with the situation, at least a reasoned clinical opinion has been offered. If the patient still has difficulty in accepting the explanation, it is not unreasonable for them to have a second opinion and a referral should therefore be made to an appropriate specialist.

No treatment with monitoring

It may be that the clinical option of (immediate or definitive) treatment is not recommended by the clinician but, rather that monitoring is considered appropriate. This may be the case for a patient who is nearing the edentulous state, i.e. they still have a few teeth that may be contributing to the stability of a partial denture. In such cases the dentist may be unsure of the outcome of treatment and may elect to recommend the status quo. The health of the remaining teeth may, however, deteriorate, and a review is therefore advisable to maintain patient comfort and also to determine whether the patient should be rendered edentulous. Similarly, if there is a possibility of an adverse reaction to a denture base material, this should be monitored and treated prior to the commencement of treatment.

Patient/mouth preparation

Occasionally, preparation of the patient or the mouth is needed if a more predictable result is to be achieved. Such situations may be for the following reasons:

- **Patients who have a gagging response**. The use of desensitisation programmes may be a protracted way of managing the problem but may enable the patient to be more empowered. Where such techniques fail, treatment may require other management techniques, such as referral to a psychologist or a hypnotherapist. Treatment options for patients with retching or gagging problems were reviewed by Barsby (1994), for example toothbrushing techniques to desensitise, temporal tamponade, breathing control and the use of training plates (see Case Study 3).
- **Problems of denture-supporting tissues: knife-shaped ridges, flabby or irregular ridges and denture granulomas**. The most

appropriate management of a patient presenting with knife-shaped and/or flabby ridges is for an appropriate impression technique to be used. In the case of denture granulomas, the patient should be advised to leave the denture out as much as possible. The condition may also be improved via gentle massage of the affected tissues (by the patient) using toothpaste, for example. Also, the use of a tissue conditioner in the existing denture may facilitate resolution. Surgical intervention may sometimes be needed, but should not be considered as first-line management, as was once the case.
- **Oral mucosal lesions**. White patches, redness, dryness and ulcers make a referral to a specialist in oral medicine appropriate. In cases of ulceration it is commonly accepted that if an ulcer is still present 1 week after the patient has left the denture out, a referral should be made for assessment of potential neoplasia. Although the dentist may feel reticent about making a referral for what appears to be a 'denture ulcer', it is better to refer than to realise that a cancer has gone undetected for six months.

Modification of the existing dentures

As was discussed earlier, modification of the existing dentures may result in more problems than the patient presented with; for example, if any expected improvements do not result, or the situation is made even worse, a successful outcome may not be achieved. It is for this reason that relines/rebases are to be discouraged as easy options. An obvious exception is the modification of immediate complete dentures during the first few months of placement.

Provisional/transitional dentures

There is merit in considering the use of provisional/transitional dentures. For the patient nearing the edentulous state there is no way to predict how well he/she will eventually cope with complete dentures. 'Training plates' permit an

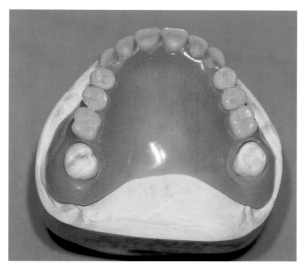

Fig. 2.2 An isthmus of silicone rubber is used to obtain a seal around a remaining tooth.

assessment of this without recourse to wholesale extractions, and allow treatment either to progress should they be tolerated or, alternatively, treatment progression to be halted should they not.

Transitional dentures have the benefit of allowing the patient to accommodate to the prosthesis/es and also to permit tooth additions as necessary. The progression from the dentate to the edentulous state can therefore be made in a less dramatic fashion.

Teeth may also be maintained and techniques used to affect a peripheral seal using a resilient material that encircles existing teeth. Such a case is illustrated in Figure 2.2.

Another form of transitional denture is illustrated in Case Study 2. Here, the current dentures are exceedingly worn. Conventional replacement dentures might potentially cause embarrassment owing to a dramatic change in appearance. The use of intermediate or transitional dentures would enable a subtle restoration to appropriate facial appearance to be realised without causing social embarrassment.

Immediate dentures

In an ideal world there would be no immediate dentures made. There is no way, other than with the use of transitional dentures, of preparing a patient for the potential problems associated with complete denture wearing. However well the dentist informs the patient of the likely end scenario, in the experience of the authors the situation is invariably traumatic for both the patient and the dentist. Advice sheets are available for patients from a variety of sources, and one such is shown in Figure 2.3. An example of the stages of this treatment is illustrated in Case Study 7.

Replica or template dentures

As has been stated previously, there is much merit in utilising the form of a patient's current dentures when the patient is able to demonstrate proficient neuromuscular control of her/his dentures; here the polished surfaces need to be templated or replicated. There is no doubt that the use of replicas has a prominent place in the management of edentulous patients, but this technique is demanding of clinical and technical skills and is not an easy option. Replica techniques have a role for the following cohort of patients:

- Where the patient requests that a spare denture is made
- Where the neuromuscular control of the patient is considered to be so poor that any significant change in denture morphology may not be tolerated
- Where the only feature considered deficient in the existing denture is the poor adaptation to the denture-bearing area
- Where a replica is required to act as a template that can be modified to deal with situations such as speech problems.

The use of these techniques, however, must be questioned in the following situations:

- Where the status of the underlying tissues merits an appropriate selective-pressure impression technique
- Where the patient dislikes the form/appearance of her/his current dentures
- Where the placement of the teeth in the current denture is resulting in problems of stability.

UNIVERSITY DENTAL HOSPITAL MANCHESTER

DEPARTMENT OF PROSTHETIC DENTISTRY

Instructions to Patients Receiving Immediate Dentures

A great deal of care and skill has been used in the production of the denture(s) which you have received. To enable you to learn to use the denture(s) as quickly as possible and get the greatest benefit from them, you are asked to note the following advice: –
Immediately following removal of teeth and insertion of dentures

(1)   Do not remove the dentures yourself. Your dentist will remove them at your next appointment.

(2)   If pain occurs relief may be obtained by taking two Paracetamol tablets at not less than four-hourly intervals.

(3)   Eat only soft foods at this stage and rinse the mouth lightly after meals.

Next Appointment
This appointment will normally be arranged about twenty-four hours following the extractions. Your dentures will be removed and any treatment necessary to improve your comfort will be carried out. You will be shown how to remove and replace the dentures and your next follow-up appointment will be arranged.

Home Care
(1)   Eating may be difficult at first. Cut your food into small pieces and take your time chewing. Avoid tough and sticky foods over the learning period.

(2)   Remove your dentures and clean them after each meal. A soft brush with soap and cold water are satisfactory for cleaning. Alternatively, a proprietary denture cleaner may be used following the manufacturers' instructions. Rinse the mouth thoroughly with warm water before replacing the dentures.

(3)   Wear the dentures night and day, removing them only for cleaning. (You will be advised when you can begin to leave the dentures out at night.)

(4)   Pain and soreness sometimes occur with new dentures and adjustment may be required. Arrange an appointment to see your dentist as soon as possible. Do not attempt to adjust the dentures yourself.

(5)   Your dentures will become progressively looser as time goes by because of changes taking place in your mouth as healing proceeds. Your dentist will advise when the time has come for the dentures to be relined or remade to restore their fit.

Fig. 2.3 An example of an advice sheet for patients who are receiving an immediate denture.

Conventional dentures

Where the patient has difficulties that would not be addressed using other techniques, 'starting from scratch' is appropriate. The chapters that follow outline the many techniques used during the fabrication of conventional dentures.

Implant/retained prostheses

There is an abundance of literature that suggests that optimal satisfaction with the edentulous state may be more predictably achieved using dental implants, which may offer improved support and retention for either removable or fixed prostheses. An example of a treated case is given in Case Study 6. It is not the aim of this book to discuss in depth the implant techniques used in dentistry.

In summary, the need for appropriate decision-making is essential so that successful treatment provision may be made.

REFERENCES

Anusavice KJ. Decision analysis in restorative dentistry. J Dent Educ 1992; 56: 812–822

Appelbaum M. Plans of occlusion. Dent Clin North Am 1984; 28:273–276

Barsby MJ. The use of hypnosis in the management of 'gagging' and intolerance to dentures. Br Dent J 1994; 176:97–102

Grant AA, Heath JR, McCord JF. Complete prosthodontics – problems, diagnosis and management. London: Mosby, 1994

McCord JF, Grey NJA, Winstanley RB, Johnson AA. A clinical overview of removable prostheses: 1. Factors to consider in planning a removable partial denture. Dent Update 2002; 29:376–381

3 Impression-making in complete dentures

The preceding chapters have emphasised the need for careful assessment and decision-making in complete denture therapy. Once a decision has been made to provide complete dentures it will be necessary, at some point, to obtain casts of the mouth to allow dentures to be constructed (away from the patient) in the dental laboratory.

This requires that impressions of the mouth be taken, from which accurate casts are produced. In order to design dentures appropriately it is necessary to obtain casts that represent the whole of the potential denture-bearing area.

ANATOMICAL EXTENT OF IMPRESSIONS

The edentulous mouth is characterised by a number of anatomical landmarks that are crucial in determining the extent of the coverage of denture-bearing tissues by complete dentures. Clinicians should be familiar with these landmarks and able to relate them to the design of complete dentures; these landmarks are listed in Table 3.1.

MAKING COMPLETE DENTURE IMPRESSIONS

It is usual for complete denture impressions to be recorded in two distinct yet related phases (Smith et al. 1999), namely primary and definitive. Each phase has different objectives:

- Primary impressions aim to record the entire denture-bearing area and thus outline the available support for a denture.

Table 3.1 Summary of anatomical extent of complete denture impressions (based on BSSPD Guidelines, Ogden 1996)

Extent of maxillary impression	Extent of mandibular impression
Residual ridges, tuberosities and hamular notches Functional width and depth of labial and buccal sulci, including frena Hard palate and its junction with the soft palate	Residual ridges and retromolar pads Functional labial and buccal sulci, (including frena and external oblique ridges) Lingual sulci, lingual frenum, mylohyoid ridges and retromylohyoid areas. (The impression should be made with the mylohyoid muscle in a raised position for the definitive impression)

- Definitive or secondary impressions aim to produce the form and extent of the fitting surface of the denture, thus maximising support, retention and stability.

Impression-making

Given the contribution that the impression surfaces of dentures make in determining patient comfort, together with functional stability and retention of complete dentures, it is important that clinicians become proficient at impression-making. For reasons of clarity, the following section will be subdivided in order to guide the reader through what may sometimes be a confusing choice of impression materials and techniques.

Common to all impression techniques is the need to ensure that the patient is comfortable and that the operator is positioned so that he/she maintains control over the flow and positioning of the impression.

Some patients are anxious about the impression-making process, and they should be given reassurance and a brief description of the process itself, together with encouragement as the visit continues.

Patients who exhibit an exaggerated gag reflex may require modification of the conventional techniques together with adjunctive therapy appropriate to their individual circumstances. This might include sedative techniques, e.g. relative analgesia, hypnosis and, potentially, acupuncture (Fiske, Dickinson 2001). The following descriptions apply to patients who do not exhibit an exaggerated gag reflex and in whom impressions have been undertaken previously without the need for adjunctive treatment.

Primary impressions

Prior to recording the impression, thought should be given to the selection of appropriate impression trays and materials. Impression trays are rigid containers used to carry the impression material into the mouth. They also support it while it sets or hardens, and subsequently during removal from the mouth and when casts are poured.

A wide selection of stock impression trays is available in metal or plastic (Fig. 3.1), and

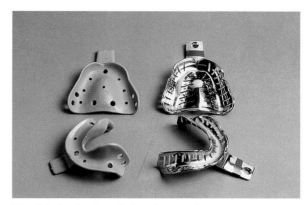

Fig. 3.1 A selection of edentulous stock trays.

selection should be based on the rigidity of the tray material plus the need to accommodate an appropriate amount of impression material and to extend to the anatomical landmarks outlined previously (Table 3.1).

Metal trays tend to come in a wider range of sizes and possess superior rigidity to plastic trays. These properties should be balanced against the need to clean and sterilise metal trays before reuse. Plastic trays are, however, intended to be disposable, and therefore infection control considerations may favour their use over metal trays.

In addition to choosing the impression tray there is also the need to select the most appropriate material with which to make the impression. The material selected should allow the use of a simple and quick technique which is capable of displacing tissues sufficiently to permit recording of the entire denture-bearing area while at the same time minimising patient discomfort.

Commonly used materials are impression compound, irreversible hydrocolloid (alginate) and silicone putty. It is possible to make an acceptable impression in any of these materials, assuming that the tray is of the correct size and the operator exercises sufficient skill and care in handling the patient, the tray and the materials used. However, alginate materials, when used together with inappropriately extended trays, are prone to result in poorly extended primary impressions, especially of the mandibular arch (Basker et al. 1993) (Fig. 3.2). Once the tray and

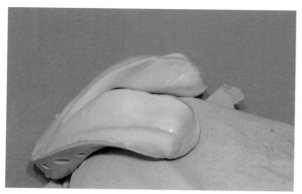

Fig. 3.2 This mandibular impression is not adequately extended in the lingual sulcus.

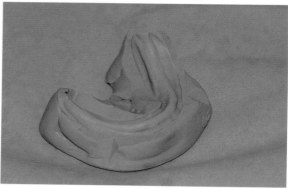

Fig. 3.3 The impression surface of the denture has been recorded in polyvinyl siloxane putty and this serves as a primary cast.

material have been chosen, the clinician should ensure that the patient has been appropriately positioned in the dental chair. It is helpful to both patient and operator if the empty impression tray is repositioned in the mouth prior to loading with the impression material, as this allows rehearsal of the positioning of the impression and familiarises the patient with the process. Once the impression material of choice has been softened/mixed as appropriate, the tray should be loaded to permit sufficient impression material to flow and extend to the anatomical features described above. It is important that the tray is not over-loaded, as this could increase patient discomfort; nor should it contain insufficient material, which would lead to an underextended impression.

Whether the maxillary or the mandibular impression is recorded first is a matter for the clinician to decide; however, as most patients are more fearful of the maxillary impression it could be argued that in most cases it is preferable that the mandibular one is made first. Then, hopefully, as patient and operator confidence increases, the potentially more troublesome maxillary impression may be made.

When the mandibular impression is being recorded the clinician should normally be positioned in front and to one side of the patient; the loaded tray should be centred over the ridge and seated so that the impression material extends beyond the periphery of the tray to fill the functional width of the sulci.

For the maxillary impression the clinician should be positioned behind the patient, as this affords more control over the upper tray and hence flow of material. It also allows the patient's head to be leaned forward should they experience nausea during the impression procedure. Once impressions have been made they should be removed from the mouth and subjected to an appropriate means of decontamination before being sent to the dental laboratory. The patient should be allowed to rinse their mouth if they so wish, as this improves their comfort.

Alternatively – and if the current dentures are perceived to have acceptable fit of the impression surfaces – this surface of the denture may be recorded in polyvinyl siloxane putty, and this would serve as a primary cast (Fig. 3.3).

Definitive impressions

These should be accurate representations of the tissues of the denture-bearing areas, together with the functional width and depth of the sulci. Definitive impressions therefore pay a crucial part in the provision of stable and retentive complete dentures (Jacobson & Kroll 1983).

As definitive impressions need to cater for a range of oral conditions that may be encountered clinically, different approaches and combinations of material have been developed to cope with this range. In certain circumstances there is a need to employ a special combination of impression trays and materials to record the supporting tissues in a particular state of displacement.

In most cases, however, a conventional approach to impression-making fulfils the requirements that have been outlined for successful definitive impressions. In all instances the manipulation and seating of the impression in the mouth are similar to those already described for primary impressions, differences being confined to the design of the individual tray and the amount and type of impression material used.

Conventional definitive impressions

The definitive impression makes use of 'special' or customised trays which have normally been constructed to the prescription of the clinician on the primary casts – specific for each patient. When prescribing special trays, the clinician needs to bear in mind the following aspects of design:

- **Peripheral extension**. The tray should cover the entire denture-bearing area within the anatomical limits previously described.
- **Material**. This should be safe to handle, compatible with biological tissues and impression materials and sufficiently rigid to preclude distortion.
- **Handles**. These should be positioned and formed so as to avoid encroaching on the surrounding tissues: for example, inappropriately designed handles may lead to distortion of the labial aspects of impressions as a result of distortion of the sulcular tissues.
- **Space for impression material**. Trays should accommodate the optimum thickness of the chosen impression material.

Examples of appropriately designed conventional special trays are illustrated in Figure 3.4a and b. One important point to note is that impression trays for complete dentures are requested without perforations so that peripheral seal can be estimated – something that is impossible with perforated trays.

Thus the clinician should have determined the type of impression technique and material to be used prior to the construction of trays, as this will determine the design of the individual trays (Table 3.2).

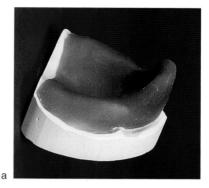

a

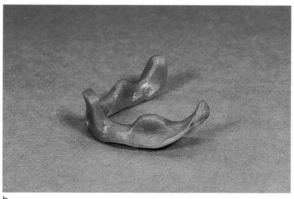

b

Fig. 3.4 (a) Maxillary special tray. (b) Mandibular special tray.

Conventional definitive impression techniques

The technique adopted by the clinician should normally follow the sequence below:

- Checking and modification of the special trays to ensure that they are appropriately extended (Fig. 3.5).
- Establishing the peripheral form of the trays in order to record the functional width and of the sulci. This normally involves the addition of thermoplastic tracing compound to the periphery of the impression tray (Fig. 3.6). If this has been done successfully in a non-perforated tray it should exhibit adequate retention.
- The tray is loaded with sufficient impression material and the denture-bearing tissues are recorded together with the functional depth of the sulci (the width has already been determined by the tracing compound). The material to be used is largely a matter of personal choice

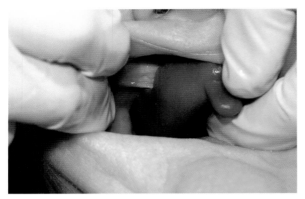

Fig. 3.5 Assessment of the maxillary special tray for appropriate extension in the sulci.

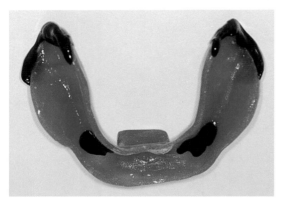

Fig. 3.6 Greenstick tracing compound added to the periphery of the denture. Anterior spacing is also seen on the impression surface anteriorly.

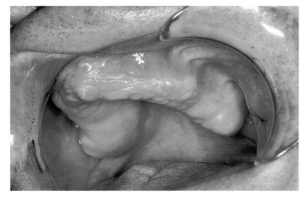

Fig. 3.7 The undercut anterior ridge plus the posterior undercuts clearly demanded that an elastic impression material be used.

by the clinician involved, the exception being the need to use an elastic material when undercut residual ridges are present (Fig. 3.7).

As has already been outlined, the state of the residual ridges, or a particular prosthodontic approach to treatment, may require the use of impression techniques that vary from the conventional approach described above. These could be considered as 'special' situations and will be described below.

Specific impression techniques

These may be required in the following circumstances:

- Displaceable ('flabby') maxillary ridge
- Fibrous mandibular ridge that has not been utilised for support ('unemployed ridge')
- Flat lower ridge covered by atrophic mucosa
- Reline impressions
- Functional, e.g. denture space ('neutral zone') and 'functional' reline impressions
- Replica/template technique – this is illustrated in Case Study 1.

As the techniques and materials differ depending on the specific technique being used, they will be considered separately in the sections that follow.

Displaceable maxillary ridge

This should have been identified during the initial assessment by palpation of the residual edentulous ridges. The extent of the displaceable tissue should be carefully determined to elicit whether firm supporting ridges are available in more posterior maxillary areas. The technique described here aims to utilise the firmer tissues, which are more likely to be capable of denture support, while reducing the pressure on the more displaceable ridge areas, hence the term selective pressure applied to this impression technique.

The impression tray should be designed with special emphasis on the location of the handle(s) and the amount of spacing for impression material. For convenience, stub handles should be sited over areas of firm tissue and not over 'flabby' areas, lest this interferes with any subsequent modification of the individual tray. As was stated previously, the tray should not be perforated by

Table 3.2 Summary of common definitive impression techniques

Impression material	Tray spacing	Notes
Irreversible hydrocolloid	3 mm	Useful when undercuts are present. Susceptible to distortion; preferably cast immediately
Zinc oxide–eugenol	Close fitting	Accurate in thin section, reduced bulk of material, rigid distorts on removal from undercuts. Potentially irritant to the tissues
Polyvinylsiloxanes	Spacing depends on viscosity	Choice of viscosities to suit clinician's preference, dimensionally stable, delayed pouring of casts possible. NB: If the existing denture is used as a 'primary tray' then at least a medium-bodied material should be used. Putty mix for template primary impression
Polyethers	2–3 mm	Hydrophilic, prone to distort if wet, careful decontamination protocol required
Polysulphides	2–3 mm	Accurate material but lengthy setting time

the technician as it is important that the clinician is able to assess the adequacy of peripheral seal following border moulding, which precedes the selective pressure impression itself (Fig. 3.8).

Once border moulding has been completed the tray should be loaded with the impression material (e.g. medium-bodied elastomer) and a maxillary impression made as previously described, with firm pressure being applied to the carefully sited stub handles. When this has been removed from the mouth and inspected to ensure acceptability, a window of impression material, together with tray, is removed in the region of the displaceable tissue (Fig. 3.9). The impression is replaced in the mouth and stabilised in position with firm upwards pressure. A low-viscosity impression material (e.g. low-viscosity elastomer) is then placed over the tissue exposed through the window in the tray (Fig. 3.10). This completes the impression, which is removed and inspected prior to decontamination using an accepted protocol before despatch to the dental laboratory.

Unemployed mandibular ridge
The initial assessment should have revealed those cases that exhibit this clinical situation. Intraoral inspection will have revealed a narrow, thread-like residual ridge that is easily displaced in a lateral

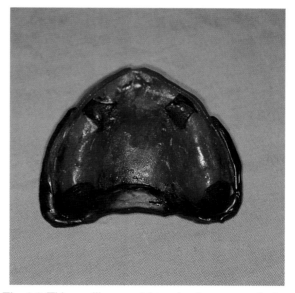

Fig. 3.8 This maxillary special tray has been customised to obtain a peripheral seal. Spacing has been provided for the impression material with tracing compound.

direction on palpation. The dental history may also suggest this condition, particularly in a patient who has attended with a lower denture packed with wet cotton wool in an attempt to improve comfort (Fig. 3.11). This technique aims

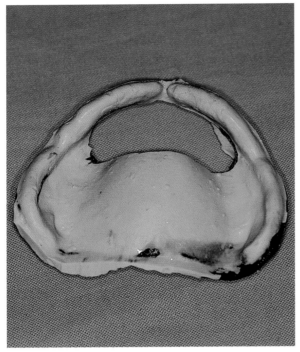

Fig. 3.9 A window equivalent to the area of displaceable tissue has been cut out.

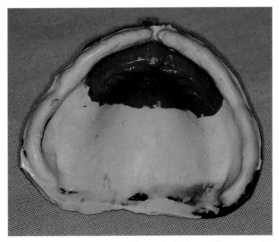

Fig. 3.10 Completed impression of displaceable area using a low-viscosity PVS.

to use the peripheral tissues, particularly the 'buccal shelves', for support, while reducing the pressure on the ridge tissues that are less capable of accepting loading.

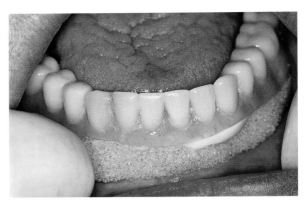

Fig. 3.11 The patient has relieved this denture with cotton wool and some foam material.

A mandibular special tray is used which has 2 mm spacing and stub handle(s), preferably sited bilaterally to avoid any areas overlying the unemployed ridge. This tray is loaded entirely with sufficient softened greenstick impression compound in order to allow a complete impression of the denture-bearing tissues to be made. Once the greenstick has hardened the impression is removed from the mouth and modified as follows. The impression compound is removed from the tray in those areas overlying the fibrous tissue, using either a heated instrument or a slowly rotating bur of appropriate dimensions. The tray is then perforated over the ridge crest (Fig. 3.12) and loaded with a fluid impression material, such as a low-viscosity elastomer or zinc oxide–eugenol paste, which is used to complete the impression (Fig. 3.13). The loaded tray is then placed in the mouth and held with firm downwards pressure: it is important that the perforations are not covered by the operator's fingers, so as to allow the free escape of excess impression material, thus preventing loading of the ridge tissue. On setting the impression is removed from the mouth, inspected and decontaminated as appropriate.

Flat lower ridge with atrophic mucosa
A technique aimed at producing an appropriate impression for this clinical situation has been fully described in the literature (McCord & Tyson 1997) and is summarised below. The objectives of this technique are to use a viscous admixture

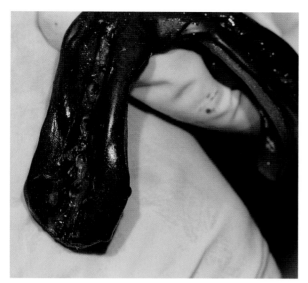

Fig. 3.12 The greenstick and the tray have been perforated over the ridge crest.

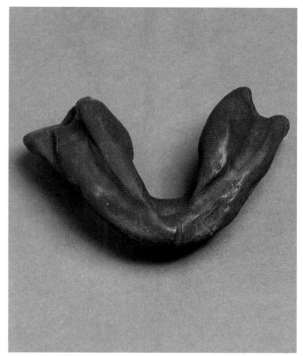

Fig. 3.14 The admix impression material has been used to record this definitive impression.

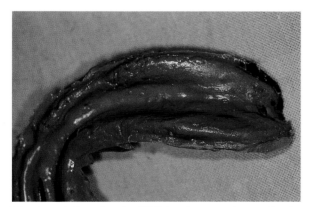

Fig. 3.13 A low-viscosity PVS has been used to make the definitive impression.

of two varieties of softened impression compound (three parts red to seven parts green) which combine to smooth soft tissue over underlying bone in an attempt to improve patient comfort (Fig. 3.14).

An individual lower tray is required which has 2 mm spacing and three stub handles, two sited in the premolar regions to act as rests for the clinician's fingers when downward seating pressure is applied and maintained while the material

hardens. A useful aspect of this technique is that it allows the fitting surface to be assessed for comfort, as the impression may be loaded via the fingers and any discomfort will be readily apparent from the patient's reaction. It is of course necessary to forewarn the patient about what is being attempted. If the patient experiences discomfort when the impression is loaded, material may be removed from the impression surface by the clinician and this process can be repeated until patient comfort has been established.

Reline/rebase impressions
As changes occur in the denture-bearing areas dentures may lose their original adaptation. When this has been recognised one clinical solution is to arrange for the denture to be relined, or in other words to have a new fitting surface to be made in the existing denture. In order to achieve this it is necessary to use the denture as an individual impression tray, in which the impression material is placed. The material chosen should

be sufficiently fluid to be able to record an impression in thin section. Important points are to ensure that the peripheries of the denture have been suitably modified where necessary by the addition of border moulding material, and also to ensure that any undercut areas are removed from the fitting surface of the denture prior to making the impression. If undercuts are not removed in this way there is a real risk of fracture of the master cast when the impression is removed. It is also critical to ensure that occlusal relationships have not been disturbed by the reline impression, and therefore the occlusion should be checked for adequacy before the impression is made and the dentures should remain in occlusal contact while the material is setting (Fig. 3.15).

Functional impressions

Functional reline The aim of this technique is to record the denture-supporting tissue in a state of functional stress. The difficulties encountered are to identify a suitable functional impression material and the appropriate length of time that the material should be used. Ideally the chosen material should flow and retain the new form (i.e. not recover). A material that has proved useful in the hands of the authors is visco-gel, which when mixed to a thick paste and placed on the fitting surface for between 2 and 4 hours produces an acceptable impression surface for the purposes of relining (Fig. 3.16).

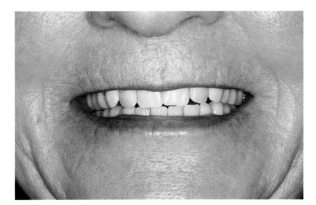

Fig. 3.15 The opposing denture is in occlusion in the recording of a reline impression.

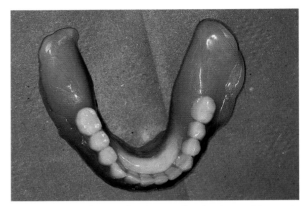

Fig. 3.16 This denture has been relined using a thixotropic material (viscous visco-gel) to give a functional reline impression.

Denture space determination This technique is well known and well established and aims to improve denture stability (invariably the lower one) by positioning the artificial teeth and polished surfaces in harmony with the action of the muscles surrounding the denture space. It has particular value in patients who experience difficulty tolerating or controlling lower dentures, especially those who have come to wear complete dentures for the first time late in life. Below is an outline of one such technique that has been used by the authors with some success.

- Complete the stages up to and including jaw registration as usual.
- Prescribe an upper wax trial as normal, but in the lower jaw request an acrylic base to which is attached a crimped length of thick wire running from molar to molar region. This is set at the previously determined occlusal vertical dimension (Fig. 3.17).
- The lower base is loaded with a mixture of tissue conditioner (e.g. visco-gel) of such a consistency that it is able to maintain form without slumping.
- The loaded lower tray is placed in the patient's mouth and the patient is instructed to swallow and make various functional movements, such as phonetics and pursing the lips. These movements indicate where inward and outwardly directed muscular activities are in equilibrium (Fig. 3.18).

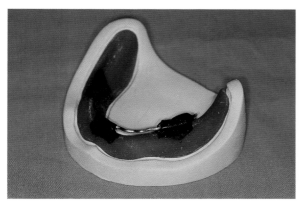

Fig. 3.17 Subframe on which the denture space determination is obtained.

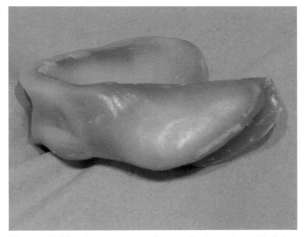

Fig. 3.18 The denture space (zone of minimal conflict) has been recorded.

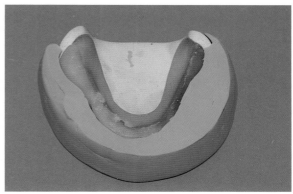

a

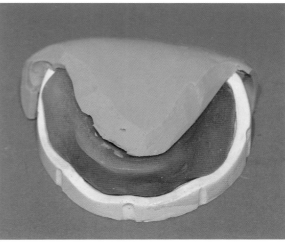

b

Fig. 3.19 (a) PVS putty has been used instead of plaster to form the labial buccal keys. (b) PVS putty has been used instead of plaster to form the lingual key.

On conclusion of the clinical procedure, the impression is decontaminated and sent to the dental laboratory together with a prescription to form plaster or PVS putty 'keys' around the buccal and lingual surfaces of the denture space impression (Fig. 3.19). The impression may then be removed from these, and when the keys are repositioned around the working cast the denture space may be poured in molten modelling wax. The teeth should be set in accordance with the denture space by reference to the aforementioned plaster 'keys'.

Although this description might suggest that it is easy to do, it is demanding both clinically and technically.

CONCLUDING REMARKS

This chapter has emphasised the need for carefully selected and executed impression techniques in the provision of stable, retentive and comfortable complete dentures. This builds upon the previously identified requirements of careful patient assessment, decision-making and clear communication between all the parties involved in complete denture provision (Table 3.3).

Table 3.3 Summary of special impression techniques

Impression technique	Impression tray	Notes
Selective pressure for displaceable maxillary ridge	Close fitting, e.g. 1 mm for elastomer (e.g. polyvinyl siloxane, PVS) impression material. Stub handles, either one at centre of palate or one on each side in the premolar/molar region, depending on tissue support	Complete impression in single phase to confirm border extension. Create window through tray and material. Make impression of displaceable tissue through window using fluid material
Unemployed mandibular ridge	2 mm spaced tray. Stub handles to avoid areas of unemployed ridge	Make impression in greenstick initially. Then relieve areas over unemployed ridge and perforate tray. Complete impression in fluid material
Flat lower ridge	2 mm spaced tray. Three stub handles: one midline, one each side premolar regions	Make impression in admix; 3 parts red compound 7 parts greenstick
Reline impressions	Existing denture modified at peripheries and by removal of undercuts from fitting surface. Also, greenstick should be applied to produce a peripheral seal and spacing on the impression surface for the impression material	Make impression in fluid material, e.g. zinc oxide–eugenol, medium-viscosity elastomer. Maintain occlusal relationships
Functional reline	Add functional reline to denture fitting surface	Patient uses denture for 2–4 hours, then cast is poured for new impression surface
Denture space determination ('neutral zone')	Lower acrylic base modified to support functional impression material at desired OVD	Usual clinical laboratory procedures up to and including registration stage. Functional movements mould suitable impression material placed on modified acrylic base to establish tooth position and form of polished surfaces
Replica technique	1° trays are dentate trays 2° trays are the templated trial dentures with autocured PMMA bases and occlusal surfaces and wax peripheries	1° impression material in PVS putty; 2° in light or medium-bodied PVS material

REFERENCES

Basker RM, Ogden AR, Ralph JP. Complete denture prescription – an audit of performance. Br Dent J 1993; 174: 278–284

Fiske J, Dickinson C. The role of acupuncture in controlling the gagging reflex using a review of ten cases. Br Dent J 2001; 190: 611–613

Jacobson TE, Kroll AJ. A comtemporary review of the factors involved in complete denture retention, stability and support. J Prosthet Dent 1983; 49: 5–15; 165–172; 306–313

McCord JF, Tyson KW. A conservative prosthodontic option for the treatment of edentulous patients with atrophic (flat) mandibular ridges. Br Dent J 1997; 182: 469–472

Ogden AR (ed) Guidelines in prosthetic and implant dentistry. London: Quintessence Publishing, 1996; 7–11

Smith PW, Richmond R, McCord JF. The design and use of special trays in prosthodontics: guidelines to improve clinical effectiveness. Br Dent J 1999; 187: 423–426

4 Registration stage

INTRODUCTION

Before complete dentures are constructed the clinician, with the aid of the technician, must build a pro-forma or template of the intended denture using – usually – wax rims. This is called the registration stage and is often perceived to be the most clinically demanding.

According to the *Glossary of Prosthodontic Terms* (Academy of Prosthodontics 1994), the registration is 'a record made of the desired maxillomandibular relationship and is used to relate casts to an articulator'. A maxillomandibular relationship record is also defined as 'a relationship of the maxilla to the mandible; any one of the infinite relationships of the mandible to the maxilla'.

In essence, the clinician is required to achieve reproducible relationships of the mandible to the maxilla (in both sagittal and coronal planes) at an appropriate vertical dimension for each patient. The importance of this factor, relevant to each patient, is addressed in an earlier chapter.

In simple terms, the registration phase may be seen as a three-dimensional prescription whereby the template of the intended denture is 'prescribed and fashioned' clinically before being dispatched to the laboratory for the placement of teeth on the trial dentures.

Prior to this stage, definitive impressions were recorded; into these, die materials are subsequently poured to make the master models. On these, bases of wax, thermoplastic resin or (poly)methylmethacrylate (PMMA) are laid and wax is poured into the land area and fashioned to create the rim (Figs 4.1 and 4.2), which is the basic form used to fashion the replacement denture.

Table 4.1 lists some of the materials that may be used as bases for record rims, with indications of effectiveness. In general, bases for occlusal

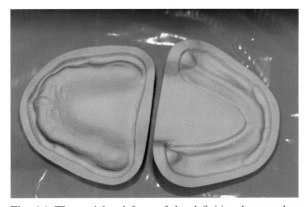

Fig. 4.1 The peripheral form of the definitive dentures has been reproduced on these casts.

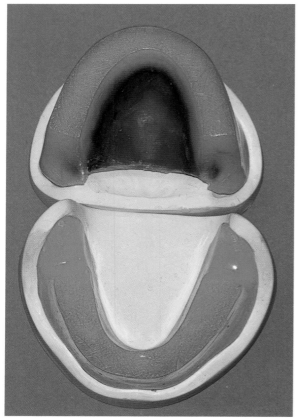

Fig. 4.2 The base material and wax have been adapted appropriately.

rims/aesthetic control bases should be (Watt & MacGregor 1986, Grant et al. 1994):

- Well adapted and conform closely to the master cast
- Stable, both on the cast and *in situ*
- Free of voids or surface projections on the impression surface
- No more than 1 mm thick over the residual ridge to prevent the base interfering with the placement of the denture teeth
- 2 mm thick in the postdam area of the maxillary denture (and 2 mm thick in the lingual flange of the mandibular denture) to impart rigidity
- Easily removed from the cast
- Smooth and rounded so as to reproduce the contours of the master cast

- Constructed in materials that are dimensionally stable at mouth temperature
- Clear of frena/muscle attachments, as this will affect stability of the rim/denture.

As wax bases per se do not provide stability, their usage is not encouraged as they may be prone to distortion. Thermoplastic resins tend to be brittle and, as they lack the versatility of PMMA, they no longer enjoy widespread usage in clinical or laboratory practice. The type of PMMA used is a matter of choice between technician and clinician, and may be autopolymerised, light polymerised or heat polymerised; the principal difference will be cost, although they vary in their levels of tissue fit. In theoretical terms, however, the heat-polymerised bases are perceived to be superior (Morris 1988).

Although this stage is often referred to as 'the bite', we would suggest that this term be abolished; rather, there are three separate but related functions to be performed in this visit. These are:

- Fashioning the labial, buccal and palatal surfaces of the maxillary rim to the desired shape for the maxillary denture
- Relating the mandible to the maxilla appropriate for each patient
- Determining the moulds and shade(s) of the teeth to be used in the dentures.

These components of conventional replacement dentures will now be considered separately; the stages for copy or template dentures, although essentially similar, will be dealt with in Case Study 1. Where possible, the evidence base for treatment stages will be supplied.

Fashioning the labial, buccal and palatal surfaces of the maxillary rim to the desired shape for the maxillary denture

This section addresses the problems of how the clinician may develop and customise the upper wax rim to the intended form of the replacement prosthesis. This cannot be done arbitrarily, but rather is achieved after a thorough assessment

Table 4.1 Common materials used as bases for record rims

Classification of base	Material	Advantages	Disadvantages
'Temporary' bases	a. Thermoplastic resin	Cheap, easy to adapt to cast, easy to adapt to postdam on master cast	Brittle, may fracture in clinical use
	b. Autopolymerised PMMA	Cheap, technicians familiar with usage	Acceptable material but handling problems possible
	c. Light-cured PMMA	Easy to make tray, quick technique	Problems of adherence of wax to base, polishing more difficult than (b) (above).
(EVA)	d. Vacuum-formed		Requires thermal vacuum machine
	e. Baseplate wax	Fast, quite cheap, not messy, easy to adapt	Easily distorted
'Permanent' bases	a. Processed resin	Rigid, accurate and stable bases – become part of final denture	Destroys master cast, good clinical and technical techniques required
	b. Cast alloys, e.g. gold, cobalt–chromium	Bases are rigid, stable and should have accurate fit	Cost more than other types, especially gold alloys. Sound impression techniques required, especially in postdam area. NB a conventional wax try-in should be performed first to establish the planned positions of the denture teeth.

of the intraoral and facial tissues, in addition to paying attention to the views of the patient and his/her expectations.

In clinical practice it is customary for the clinician to receive maxillary wax rims, which are duly moulded into the form of the upper denture at the chairside. The form of the maxillary wax rim or block depends, essentially, on how the technicians were taught. There is probably considerable variation among technicians with regard to the positioning of the labial face of the rim. The consequence of this is that it is often a matter of chance that wax has to be removed or added to the upper rim. In an attempt to save clinical time, and at the same time render the maxillary rims more appropriate in form for each patient, two techniques have evolved: the biometric technique and the Swissedent technique. Both will be described for interested practitioners and their technicians, as they both have the theoretical advantage of saving chairside time. There may be other techniques, but these two are perhaps the best known.

The biometric principle

Watt and MacGregor (1986) advocated these guidelines in an attempt to help the clinician take account of changes in facial profile that occurred subsequent to the loss of teeth, predominantly in the maxilla. They recommended that the maxillary denture teeth be placed in their mean pre-extraction positions; these average values cited by Watt and MacGregor were determined over a 30-month period in a group of patients who had been rendered edentulous. The provision

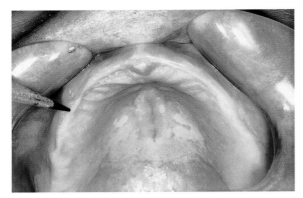

Fig. 4.3 The cord-like structure indicated is termed the lingual gingival margin.

of reference points is problematic in edentulous patients, and the midpalatal areas have been cited as 'fixed areas'. Watt and MacGregor also stated that the remnants of the (maxillary) lingual gingival margin (LGM, Fig. 4.3) were valid points to use for reference. Average values for maxillary teeth of replacement dentures are shown in Table 4.2.

This technique has several advantages, in that it could be a useful guideline for the placement of denture teeth into what was approximately the position of the natural teeth. A second potential advantage is the resultant placement of the maxillary (denture) teeth labial/buccal to the residual ridge. This would naturally result in greater inherent stability for the mandibular denture by virtue of the palatal cusps of the posterior maxillary teeth occluding into the central fossae of

the posterior mandibular teeth, thereby directing occlusal forces on to the residual ridge. This positioning of the mandibular molar teeth over the residual mandibular ridge (and assuming that teeth of appropriately narrow buccolingual width are chosen) tends to avoid constriction of tongue space.

It is accurate to state that this treatment philosophy does not enjoy universal use. One reason for this could be that it does not necessarily customise the denture form for each patient, nor does it cater for biological ageing, as it assumes that there is a normal distribution of residual ridge resorption – which there most certainly is not. A second problem with this philosophy is that anatomical features not dissimilar to the remnants of the lingual gingival margin have been observed in patients suffering from anodontia.

The other system referred to, the Swissedent system, will be summarised later.

The clinical stages recommended for the registration stage, therefore, are as follows.

General assessment prior to placement in the patient's mouth

Unless the clinician has cast the definitive impression and has scored the master cast to define the postdam, the rim will not exhibit a clinically meaningful peripheral seal. This may be achieved by the technician relieving the master cast with wax (1 mm thick) but placing this relief 2 mm short of the vibrating line, thereby incorporating a form of postdam inherent in the denture base. The clinician must be aware, however, that this would not conform to the anatomy of the tissues comprising the patient's postdam (Fig. 4.4). It would, however, provide an acceptable peripheral seal as long as the functional width and depth of the sulci were faithfully restored in wax.

At the registration visit, the clinician should score the postdam area of the master cast to demonstrate the depth of postdam required for each patient. The posterior border of the upper denture should displace the mucosa overlying the aponeurosis of tensor palati at the junction between the hard and soft palates. As the details of the displaceability of the tissues of the postdam are known only to the clinician, it is his/her

Table 4.2 Average values of maxillary labial/buccal bone loss following loss of teeth. The values in the right-hand column indicate by how much the labial/buccal faces of the maxillary rim are built out from the LGM remnants

Tooth position	Average horizontal bone loss
Incisor	6.5 mm
Canine	8.5 mm
Premolar	10.5 mm
Molar	12.5 mm

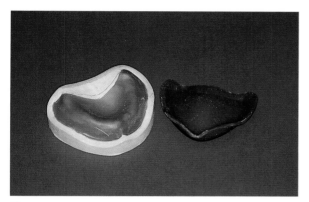

Fig. 4.4 A semblance of a postdam may be obtained by stopping a wax spacer short of the areas on the cast (corresponding to the function of the hard and soft palates) prior to applying the light-cured resin base.

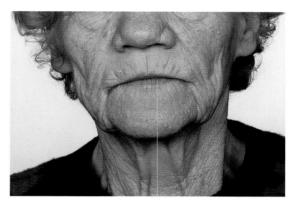

Fig. 4.6 The upper lip has been distorted by too thick a rim in the depth of the sulcus. The creation of a simian groove will affect the position of the resting maxillary lip.

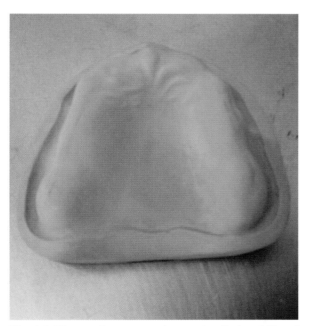

Fig. 4.5 The postdam, appropriate to the displaceability of the tissues of the patient, has been scribed. Note the extension buccal to the pterygohamular fold.

responsibility to score the appropriate extent and depth of the postdam using, for example, a Le Cron carver or similar instrument (Fig. 4.5).

After immersing the rim in disinfectant material, in keeping with conventional infection-control procedures and prior to inserting the rim into the mouth, the clinician should ensure that the rim is well adapted to the master cast. Alternating finger pressure on both sides of each rim in turn should not elicit a rocking of the rim on either cast.

When the maxillary rim has been inserted into the mouth and the clinician has ensured its stability, the first clinical step is to ensure that the infranasal tissues are harmonious with the soft tissues of the middle third of the face. Failure to do this may affect the form and length of the upper lip (Fig. 4.6) by raising it inappropriately – this may adversely influence the subsequent stages.

Confirm that the upper lip is adequately supported. This should result in restoration of the vermilion border and may result in restoration of the philtrum (it may not always be desirable or possible to restore the latter) (Fig. 4.7). Some clinical guidelines recommend that the vertical nasolabial angle should be 90°, although the lack of evidence-based studies verifying this casts doubt on this guideline (Brunton & McCord 1993).

When the upper lip has been restored appropriately for the patient, the clinician then has to determine the position of the incisal point relative to the resting upper lip. Some textbooks recommend that the incisal level of the upper rim be 2 mm inferior to the resting upper lip; this may well be appropriate for some patients but, as the relationship of the upper lip to the incisal points of the maxillary central incisor teeth varies in any

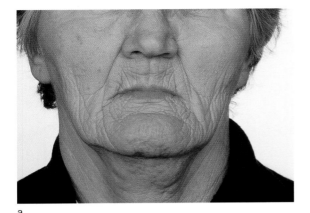

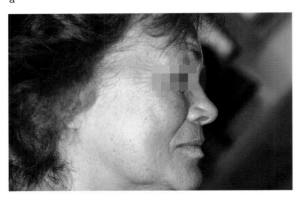

Fig. 4.7 (a) Typical unrestored edentulous upper lip. (b) Restored edentulous upper lip; note restoration of the vermilion border.

The next step in this clinical exercise is to determine the maxillary anterior plane. Given the position of the incisal point, the plane of the upper six anterior teeth is typically or conventionally determined by making it parallel to the inter-pupillary line: this may be done using a Fox's occlusal plane guide (Fig. 4.8a) or any device giving a horizontal plane, e.g. a wooden spatula. This guideline has been in the prosthodontic armoury for many years and is a useful early-learning instrument. More experienced clinicians will recognise, however, that more correctly the incisal plane should represent only the two central incisors, owing to the natural stepping of the six anterior teeth (see Chapter 5, Fig. 5.3).

When this has been performed, there is merit in determining the position of the midpoints of the

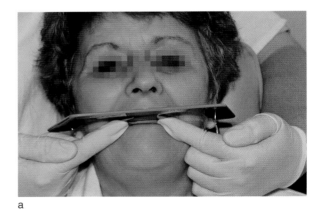

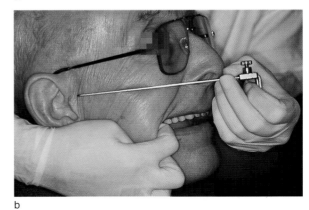

Fig. 4.8 (a) Assessment of incisal plane using a Fox's occlusal plane guide. (b) Assessment of right posterior plane using a Fox's occlusal plane guide.

one individual throughout life (McCord & Grant 2000), it is incumbent on the clinician to decide what is clinically appropriate for each patient; younger patients may reasonably be expected to show 4–5 mm of tooth beneath the resting lip, especially if they had a Class 2 division 1 profile. In contrast, a 70-year-old patient might more appropriately have the incisal point level with the resting lip, or possibly 1 mm above it.

The above relates to the vertical positioning of the incisal points. Anteroposterior verification of the placement of the incisal point may be achieved by asking the patient to say a word containing a fricative consonant (labiodental sound), e.g. 'fish'; in general terms, the incisal point should correspond to the vermilion border of the lower lip (McCord et al. 1994).

maxillary canine teeth. One useful way to record this is to use a photograph of the patient when he/she was dentate. A clear, face-on photograph is required for this, but regrettably these are not always available. Using the pupils as stable reference points, the clinician may determine the relative position of the upper canine teeth using the ratio:

$$\frac{\text{Actual interpupillary distance}}{\text{Actual intercanine tip distance}} = \frac{\text{Photographic interpupillary distance}}{\text{Photographic intercanine distance}}$$

A second useful technique is to extend dental floss from the inner canthus of the eye, via the lateral border of the alar cartilage (with the patient smiling) on to the incisal edge of the maxillary rim (Fig. 4.9).

Using the canine points on the maxillary rim as reference points, the right and left posterior planes are formed. The accepted guideline is that this plane is parallel to the line drawn from the inferior border of the alar cartilage to a position two-thirds of the way up the tragus (Fig. 4.8b).

Using the mark on the rim corresponding to the canine tips as a reference point, the buccal form of the maxillary rim may be moulded by reducing the inferior borders of the posterior rims by 3–5°. This procedure creates what are known as the buccal corridors and creates a more natural smile (Fig. 4.10).

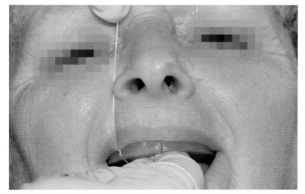

Fig. 4.9 Useful guide to positioning of the tips of the maxillary canines.

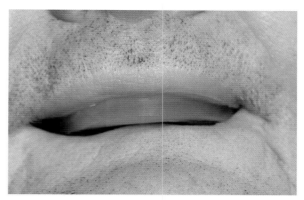

Fig. 4.10 Creation of a buccal corridor is clear on the right-hand side of this image.

Before completing the customising of the upper rim, the following should be scribed clearly on the anterior aspect of the rim (Fig. 4.11a):

- Centre line
- High smile line
- Canine points.

In addition to serving as location points for the technician to position the anterior maxillary teeth, these may be used by the clinical staff in selecting the moulds for the maxillary anterior teeth.

With the maxillary rim *in situ*, ask the patient to smile; the maxillary rim should appear to be parallel to the lower lip line when smiling (Fig. 4.11b).

Depending on the occlusal and stability requirements of the patient, the clinician may consider it necessary to use a facebow to transfer the relationship of the upper rim to an arbitrary hinge axis. Although it must be conceded that whereas it may not be strictly necessary to use a facebow in all complete maxillary denture cases, there is no valid objection to the use of the facebow transfer in the prescription of complete dentures.

The facebow transfer record

The facebow transfer, in this context, is used to transfer the relationship of the maxillary plane to the intercondylar axis on the patient. Once established, this relationship is transferred to the articulator so that the casts of the edentulous

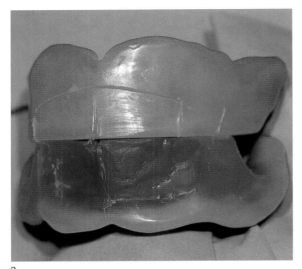

a

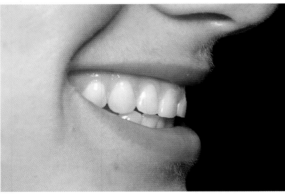

b

Fig. 4.11 (a) Salient features to be scribed on the maxillary rim. (b) Note how incisal/occlusal edges conform to lower lip form.

one other selected anterior point. In practical terms, a facebow consists of three components; a facebow fork, an anterior locator, and a U-bow used to locate the condyles (the two posterior determinants).

As was mentioned earlier, the principal purpose of the facebow is to record the relationship of the patient's maxillary plane to the patient's transverse condylar axis and then transfer that relationship to the articulator. To transfer that plane, therefore, three points must be used. Two are located posteriorly, to record the arbitrary transverse axis, and one is located anteriorly (Fig. 4.12).

We recommend the use of a facebow transfer record simply because this ensures that the plane of the maxillary complete denture will be better aligned to the condyles and hence the mandibular arch during mandibular movements. This is particularly important when complete maxillary dentures are opposed by a natural dentition (or a natural dentition plus a lower partial denture), when displacing forces on the maxillary denture may be profound. Without the facebow transfer, technicians tend to set up the maxillary rim with the rim parallel to the worktop; this, clearly, is not the typical plane of orientation of the maxillary occlusal plane (Fig. 4.13). If the patient only exhibits vertical chewing movements, then this may not be a major issue and facebow transfers are not strictly necessary.

There is a range of facebows available, and the authors do not know of any evidence indicating

maxilla assume the same relationship to the articulator's intercondylar axis. For complete denture work, a hinge axis facebow which is kinematically determined is considered not required, and a simple facebow using an arbitrary axis will suffice.

In essence, a facebow is a caliper-like instrument used to record the spatial relationship of the maxillary arch to the temporomandibular joints and then transfer this relationship to an articulator; it orientates the (maxillary) dental cast in the same relationship to the opening axis of the articulator. Customarily the anatomic references are the mandibular condyles' transverse axis and

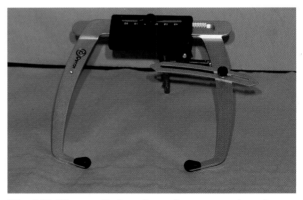

Fig. 4.12 The transfer bow shows the two posterior reference points (plus the anterior reference point).

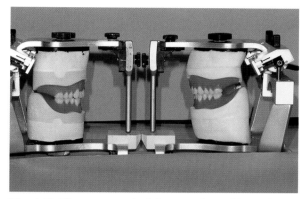

Fig. 4.13 The set-up on the left was performed by setting up parallel to the laboratory worktop; that on the right was achieved via a facebow transfer. The difference in the angulation of the planes is clear.

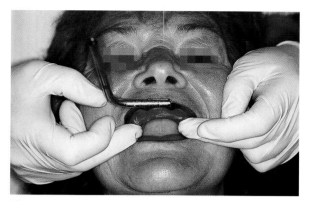

Fig. 4.14 The edentulous bite fork engages the wax of the side of the rim and does not affect the occlusal surface.

that one is better than another; we believe that practitioners should be encouraged to use the system with which they are familiar and which is compatible with the articulator used by the dental team. The system demonstrated in this book is the Denar system, and the reader will note that the posterior points are earpieces and the anterior point is located 46 mm superior to the tip of the lateral incisor tooth or its equivalent location on the maxillary rim. In fact, this measurement is arbitrary and is, in the Denar articulator, the midpoint between the upper and lower arms of the articulator; there should therefore be space in the articulator to accommodate both casts.

In all types of transfer bow for edentulous patients the bite fork of choice is an edentulous facebow, which should not therefore alter the form of the occlusal and incisal edges of the maxillary rim (Fig. 4.14).

Swissedent technique

Another technique that helps customise the maxillary rim is the Swissedent technique. This relies on close and unambiguous communication between the clinician and the technician. It uses two distinct measurements for each patient so that the upper rim (termed the aesthetic control base, ACB) may be customised for each one. These two measurements are related to the patient's facial

form and are taken immediately after the definitive impressions have been recorded, and despatched along with these impressions to the laboratory.

The first measurement is taken via what is called the papillameter (Fig. 4.15a). The procedures to be followed for the papillameter reading are:

- Place the papillameter inside the patient's upper lip and let it rest on the incisive papilla.
- Add addition-cured polyvinyl siloxane (PVS) putty to the papillameter and mould the upper lip to restore the vermilion border. In younger patients the philtrum may be restored, but this may not be possible in older patients (Fig. 4.15b).
- Determine how much of the upper incisor will be shown under the upper resting lip length (see below).
- Level the PVS at the incisal level and record the reading from the graduated scale on the papillameter (Fig. 4.15c).
- The customised papillameter is sent to the laboratory and gives the technician sufficient information to prepare an upper rim that provides upper lip support according to the judgement of the clinician. Patient information, e.g. from photographs or via dentures favoured by the patient, may also be used to help determine an upper lip form which is well perceived by the patient.
- Another instrument that could give the same result is the Alma Gauge. This consists of a

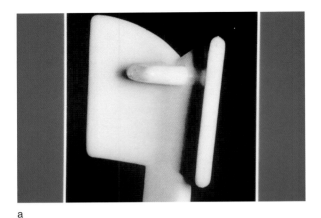

a

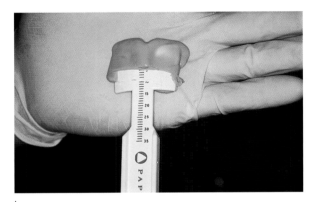

b

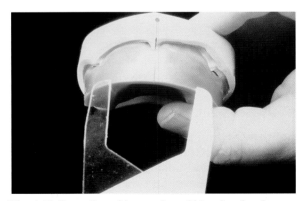

c

Fig. 4.15 (a) The papillameter – the rest on the left is to position the incisive papilla. (b) The PVS has customised the papillometer for the patient. (c) The positioning of the incisal point may be recorded.

graduated base and a spring-loaded pointer which is also graduated. The denture being 'templated' (± modification) is placed on the graduated base and the pointer placed in the impression surface of the denture in the middle of the area occupied by the incisive papilla. The distance from the pointer to the incisal tip of the central incisors may be read off the (horizontal) graduated scale on the table. The vertical distance from the pointer tip to the incisal tips is then read off the graduated scale of the pointer, giving a three-dimensional reading from the incisive papilla to the midincisal point (see Case Study 1).

The second recording concerns the anterior **width** of the upper rim, and for this a calliper-like device called an alameter is used. The alameter's use is based on a reasonable clinical guideline, namely that the width (i.e. horizontal distance) between the alar cartilages in a smiling patient is approximately equal to that of the canine tips (Fig. 4.16). This reading enables the technician to evaluate the width of the upper rim, assuming that there is symmetry about the palatal midline.

When the maxillary rim is deemed to be of an acceptable form, the clinician may then begin to relate the maxillary arch to the mandibular arch.

Fig. 4.16 Recording of intercanine width using the alameter gauge.

Relating the mandible to the maxilla appropriate for each patient

This is a very important procedure in the production of complete dentures, as errors introduced at this stage can result in dentures which are uncomfortable or unwearable, with obvious social and functional problems to the patient and perhaps medicolegal problems for the clinician. It is a *sine qua non* that intermaxillary relations are three-dimensional, namely vertical (the occlusal vertical dimension, OVD), sagittal (anteroposterior) and coronal, and each should be carefully assessed.

Vertical relationships

In the natural dentition there is a space between the occlusal surfaces of the teeth of the opposing jaws when they are at rest and with the head upright. This space – the freeway space (FWS) or interocclusal distance – is determined by a balance between the elevator and depressor muscles attached to the mandible, and the elastic nature of the surrounding soft tissue. It is usually measured indirectly by noting the difference between the resting vertical dimension (RVD) of the face using, for example, a Willis bite gauge, and subtracting from this the vertical dimension with the teeth in occlusal vertical dimension (OVD).

A similar set of circumstances is considered to exist with the edentulous patient – although the RVD may differ from that which pertained when natural teeth were present, as it is now known that the RVD is not a stable position throughout life for a given individual. The OVD, however, may be considered as a determinant as to whether a patient will be able to tolerate wearing dentures without intraoral tissue damage occurring, as well as being an important aspect of the appearance of the denture-wearing patient. For these reasons the starting point from which the OVD is estimated is the RVD (Zarb et al. 1990).

Because of the role played by the elastic properties of the soft tissue environment of the mouth, the importance of factors affecting the position of the mandible should be considered when determining the RVD. For example, the insertion of the mandibular denture or record rim prior to determining the RFH is a useful exercise, as is having the head of the patient positioned reproducibly, i.e. the head held vertically, as tilting the head backwards pulls the mandible away from the maxilla, and tilting forward tends to push the mandible and attached structures closer to the maxilla.

RVD measurement

Many methods have been advocated for the measurement of the RVD. These include various facial measurements, swallowing methods, biting force measurements, phonetic methods, tactile methods and electromyographic measurements. Clinicians are advised to use a combination of some of the above for a simplified clinical determination of RVD. The most common method is to select two measuring points in the midline of the face – typically one related to the nose and one to the chin. These points must be on sites of minimal influence from the muscles of facial expression to avoid skin movement, and should be chosen only after careful observation. The measurement is made with the patient in a relaxed and comfortable position and wearing the previously worn denture or wax rim. A Willis bite gauge (or any similar measuring device) may be used for the measurement, as it incorporates a suitable scale (Fig. 4.17).

Before recording the measurement, ask the patient to moisten his or her lips and bring them into light contact; then ask the patient to swallow and relax the jaws. Verification of the measured value can be attempted by asking the patient to say the letter 'm' while the measurement is made. The general appearance of the patient's face and its proportions should also be taken into account. Attention should be paid to any unwanted skin movement during the recording of measurements, as failure to do so may lead to erroneous results.

In conventional techniques, once the RVD has been established the maxillary and mandibular bases and rims are placed in the mouth after the upper rim has been moulded. The mandibular rim is reduced in height (usually; or added to if undersized) until it contacts the upper rim evenly

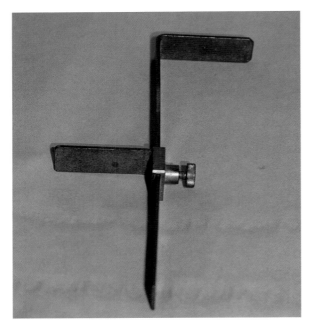

Fig. 4.17 Willis bite gauge used to record RFH.

of a freeway space effectively causes continuous clenching of the teeth. Painful mucosa over the denture-bearing areas and myalgia (typically associated with the masseter muscles) may become evident, as may symptoms suggestive of temporomandibular joint dysfunction. The teeth are liable to contact (causing clicking) during speech, and other speech problems may occur. These are generally sounds affected by an inability to approximate the lips (e.g. 'p', 'b' and 'm' sounds). Patients with inappropriately large OVDs may complain of a less than desirable appearance of their dentures ('too much tooth showing') (Fig. 4.18a).

Where the OVD is underestimated, lack of support of the angles of the mouth (causing

at a vertical dimension of occlusion some 2–4 mm less than the established RVD. This provides for a freeway space of 2–4 mm and establishes the OVD. In establishing the height of the mandibular rim, the relative height of both the maxillary and mandibular rims should be considered. As a practical consideration, an element of reasonable balance between the two rims is desirable. Excessive height of the lower rim can have the effect of 'walling in' the tongue, causing an unstable lower denture. On the other hand, insufficient depth of the lower rim can result in a denture having poor aesthetics and, further, may result in tongue biting. Conventional wisdom, however, would indicate that the occlusal plane should be below the dorsum of the tongue at rest.

Potential errors in the determination of the OVD

Provision of an appropriate OVD is important because of the consequences that can result from an over- or underestimation of this value.

The provision of an excessive vertical dimension may result in increased risk of trauma to the tissues underlying the dentures, as the absence

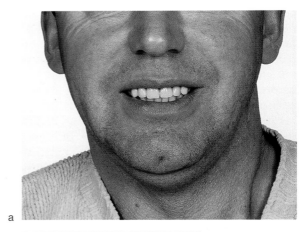

a

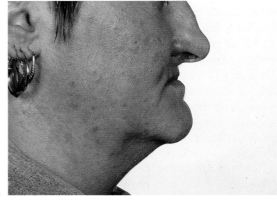

b

Fig. 4.18 (a) Inappropriately excessive OVD, seen by obvious problems in obtaining an 'unstrained' lip seal. (b) Lack of OVD has resulted in a pseudo-prognathic profile.

dribbling and possibly angular cheilitis) may be apparent. Masticatory efficiency may be reduced and, because of a lack of adequate support of the lips and cheeks, aesthetics may be poor. Mandibular protrusion on closure may also occur (Fig. 4.18b).

It should be thus apparent that careful and measured clinical judgement is required, and, furthermore, it must not be assumed that the value selected is immutable, as the generally quoted value for the freeway space (2–4 mm) is an average one and, as such, it should be appreciated that some patients may require a larger, or smaller, value, e.g. where atrophic mucosa exists in a middle-aged person an increased FWS might prevent/reduce trauma to the residual mandibular tissues (Gonzalez 1988).

There are several accepted tests that can be applied to verify the established OVD, but because during the registration stage occlusal rims are so different from the form of teeth to be used, it is very difficult to apply tests for suitability of the chosen value at this stage. Further checks on the established OVD will need to be made at the trial stage (see below).

SAGITTAL (ANTEROPOSTERIOR) RELATIONSHIPS

By virtue of the fact that it is deemed to be reproducible, the generally agreed position for recording these relationships is the retruded contact position (RCP). A second reason for recording RCP in edentulous patients is that denture stability (which may be problematic in any event) will be compromised if unbalanced contacts occur between opposing dentures as a result of the teeth, when set up, being in other than RCP, and this may have the potential to result in abnormal temporomandibular joint activity as patients attempt to accommodate to incorrect occlusal relation (Grant & Johnson 1992).

Following adjustment of the occlusal rims to the selected OVD, the rims should be inserted into the mouth and the patient persuaded to close gently with the mandible in the RCP. The word 'bite' should be avoided, as it suggests to the patient that forceful closure is required, and this might result in a recorded intermaxillary

relation which is protrusive to the most retruded position.

Several methods have been suggested to assist the patient to position the mandible in RCP; some patients have the capacity to relax the muscles attached to the mandible so that the operator can readily move the mandible up and down as it rotates about the condyles. In those circumstances the mandible is in RCP and can be guided there during the registration procedure. Other patients are able to retrude the mandible when the tongue is curled back in the roof of the mouth to feel the posterior border of the upper base, or a shallow ridge of wax placed on the palatal area of the base posterior to the first molar region. Some patients are unable to achieve this position, and it may be necessary to use a customised prosthesis such as an occlusal pivot (Case Study 2.)

Methods of registration

Recording the RCP requires that upper and lower rims be fixed in position with the mandible in its most retruded position and with the jaws separated by the established OVD.

A variety of methods for securing a record of the retruded jaw relations (RJR) have been used, with varying degrees of success.

- Wax squash bite
- Wax rims with 'Manchester' blocks
- Intraoral tracing (Gothic arch tracing).

Wax squash bite

The wax squash bite involves placing a horseshoe-shaped roll of softened wax between the maxillary and mandibular rims and having the patient close the jaws together. The mandibular rim is first reduced in height to provide space for the wax. Results using this method are unpredictable because of the lack of control of the mandible during closure, and thus in obtaining RCP. Further, this method of recording takes no account of mandibular movements other than the final act of closure – and that is uncertain (Fig. 4.19). In addition, if the wax wafer is not uniformly softened throughout its length, an unstable

Table 4.3 Guidelines to the selection and position of upper anterior teeth* indicate that photographs of appropriate quality are used

Nature of guideline	Frontal view	Sagittal view	Coronal view	Other
Pre-extraction	Photograph *Relate canine points to pupils *Relate canine points to inter alar width (smiling) *Relate six anterior teeth to smile line Cast of arch Radiograph Relative of similar facial appearance	Photograph *Relate six anterior teeth to smile line Cast of arch Radiograph Relative with similar appearance	Photograph (unlikely) Cast of arch Radiograph (unlikely) Relative with similar appearance	Extracted teeth
Post-extraction	Central incisors restore philtrum if possible Central incisors restore vermillion border Incisal points and smile line determine height of tooth (relate to age of patient) Position of canine points Relate to inter-alar width (smiling) Relate to pupils (require pre-extraction photograph) Relation of maxillary rim to smile line	Vertical nasolabial angle Amount of tooth showing below lip at rest (age-related) Relation of maxillary rim to smile line		

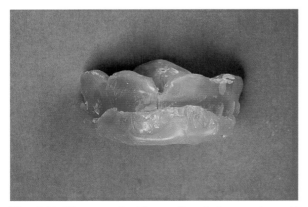

Fig. 4.19 Wax squash bites offer little certainty of reproducibility.

relationship with the underlying tissues is recorded.

Wax rims

The conventional method, which has a higher degree of success than the squash bite, also involves the use of wax interposed between the rims to secure a registration. When the maxillary rim (ACB) has been formed, and prescribed to suit the patient, the mandibular rim is placed in the mouth and trimmed until it contacts the maxillary rim evenly in RCP and at the selected OVD (Fig. 4.20). This is done by selectively removing points of first contact.

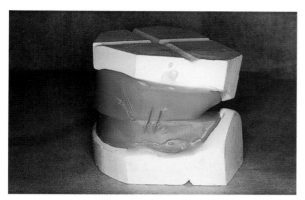

Fig. 4.20 Typical wax rims.

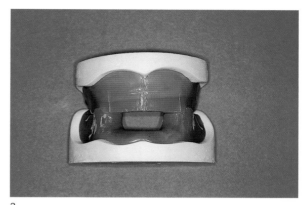

a

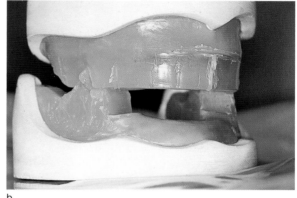

b

Fig. 4.21 (a) Manchester rims. Simplified and reduced occlusal table on the mandibular rim and a more customised maxillary rim. (b) Sealed mandibular rim.

Wax rims with Manchester blocks

These relatively large wax rims may not always give reproducible results. Even in experienced hands it is not always easy to detect premature contacts along the lengths of the rims. For this reason, we have developed a modified and simplified version of the above. This comprises a simplified mandibular rim and contains several elements incorporated to ensure that the carefully established OVD is maintained, and that the bases are maintained in stable relationship to the underlying tissues during the procedure. The lower base has, attached to it, two pillars of wax which are situated in the area onto which the second premolar/first molar teeth would be placed (Fig. 4.21a). The length of these 'pillars' is approximately 1 cm, and therefore the operator merely has to establish bilateral even contact on these pillars at the selected OVD (and then seal the rims with registration paste or other such medium).

This method, which we call the Manchester block method, provides control over the OVD, ensures a stable relationship between the bases and the underlying tissues and also provides a record which can be simply returned to the mouth to verify its accuracy. To obtain a functional impression of the labial component of the lower arch, carding wax or PVS putty may be attached to the labial aspect of the rim and a closed-mouth impression used to determine the anterior denture-spaced form (Fig. 4.21b).

The principal disadvantages of both the wax rim techniques, however, are the uncertainty of achieving a verifiable RCP (unless wax triangles are used) and the lack of information on border positions of the mandible.

Intraoral tracing

A reliable method of obtaining RCP plus a record of border positions is by means of an intraoral tracing – often referred to as the arrowhead or Gothic arch tracing.

This technique uses two pieces of apparatus, one for each arch, both mounted on rigid stable bases, usually made of light-cured PMMA. The maxillary apparatus comprises a metallic plate

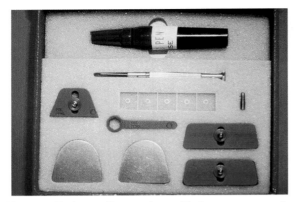

Fig. 4.22 Basic maxillary and mandibular components for recording arrowhead tracing.

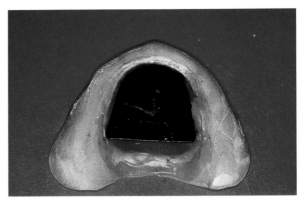

Fig. 4.23 Typical Gothic arch or arrowhead tracing.

which occupies the palatal aspect of the apparatus. The mandibular apparatus has a flat plate containing an adjustable central-bearing screw (1 mm thread) mounted on wax or compound 'pivots' added to a light-cured PMMA base (Fig. 4.22). The flat plate links the two pivots on the base. The adjustable central-bearing screw is made to contact the upper plate at right-angles and at the selected OVD. The bases are adjusted so that no contact can occur between them, and the patient can make lateral mandibular excursions with contact of the central-bearing pin on the upper plate only. The patient is requested to swallow, to indicate a central (RCP) position.

To record border positions, the patient is asked to swallow and then asked to make:

- Three protrusive movements before returning to RCP
- Three left lateral excursions and then to return to RCP
- Three right lateral excursions before returning to RCP.

The patient should then be allowed to become familiar with the two pieces of apparatus in his/her mouth and the practitioner should practise these movements before recording the tracing. This is done by coating the upper plate with, for example, ink from a felt-tipped pen and then asking the patient to replicate the protrusive and lateral movements. The alternate lateral jaw movements scribe on the upper plate two arcs of rotation,

which intersect in a position corresponding to RCP. In addition, it is from this point that the protrusive tracing commences and returns (Fig. 4.23).

To validate this position a perforated Perspex coverslip is placed with the perforation over the arrowhead and waxed in place. The patient is then asked to swallow, and confirmation of RCP is achieved by the central-bearing screw engaging the perforation (Fig. 4.24).

This fixed registration records the vertical and anteroposterior intermaxillary relations. To record the coronal relationship, plaster of Paris or PVS putty is then placed between the bases and the central-bearing screws to ensure an unambiguous relationship (Fig. 4.25).

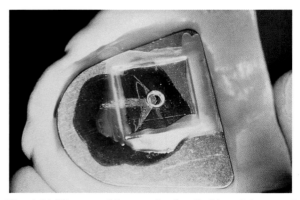

Fig. 4.24 The apex of the arrowhead or Gothic arch is covered by a Perspex disc.

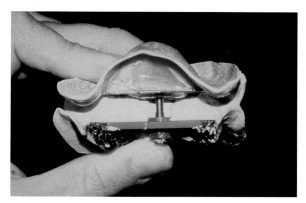

Fig. 4.25 Sealed assembly.

When these three-dimensional intermaxillary registrations have been completed, they will be sent to the laboratory along with the ACB and facebow transfer to be articulated. Although teeth have still to be selected (see below) it is appropriate to consider briefly the types of articulator on which the casts are to be mounted, as the proper adjustment of these may require additional records.

ARTICULATORS FOR COMPLETE DENTURES

The use of articulators to enhance clinical practice has been the subject of recent reviews (Cabot 1997) to which readers are referred for further information. We shall confine our discussion to simple basic points.

Articulators in common use for the production of complete dentures comprise:

- Simple hinge (plane line) articulators
- Moveable, fixed condylar path articulators
- Semiadjustable articulators.

The simple hinge articulator allows the construction only of a centric occlusion, whereas the fixed condylar path instrument allows some approximate lateral and protrusive occlusion to be developed. The semi-adjustable articulator allows the establishment of more accurate or customised lateral and protrusive as well as centric occlusion.

Few simple hinge articulators have provision for accepting a facebow record, and so this further limits their usefulness. Both the fixed condylar and the semiadjustable types will accept facebow records and, in addition, the more adjustable instruments accept protrusive and lateral interocclusal records to allow full benefit of their capability. Facebows are considered to improve the accuracy of occlusal development of these articulators (Cabot 1997).

With the maxillary cast mounted via a facebow transfer and the mandibular arch related to the maxillary arch via the Gothic arch tracing, the development of satisfactory eccentric (lateral and protrusive) occlusion and articulation is possible. In addition, small changes (2–3 mm) in the vertical dimension may be achieved on the articulator, should this be required, without a new registration being necessary.

DETERMINING THE MOULDS AND SHADE(S) OF THE TEETH TO BE USED IN THE DENTURES

The dental literature abounds with anecdotal references to the aesthetic aspects of complete denture construction. Unfortunately, no substantive evidence base has been established, and this aspect of denture provision is a mixture of pseudo-science and artistic flair, the latter being a paradigm of clinical skill, technical flourish and, most important of all, patient compliance and acceptance. The combination of science and art has led to a variety of guidelines to help the dental surgeon in the selection of (replacement) denture teeth. Unfortunately, on the evidence of prescriptions sent to dental laboratories these well-intended guidelines are often cast aside (Basker et al. 1993, Barsby et al. 1995). These studies have demonstrated that, in the majority of cases, clinicians fail to record any selection of tooth mould and/or shade for dentures; this, by implication, means that an abdication of responsibility has occurred. This omission might indicate a lack of awareness of the importance of body image to the edentulous individual and is perhaps suggestive of a diminution of the importance of complete denture prosthodontics currently. For the sake of the edentulous population, and our profession, this must not continue.

To simplify the task of selecting teeth, we recommend considering this stage of the visit as comprising four elements:

- Selection of maxillary anterior teeth
- Selection of mandibular anterior teeth
- Selection of posterior teeth types and moulds
- Selection of shade(s) of the anterior and posterior teeth.

Selection of maxillary anterior teeth

If patients have pre-extraction records (e.g. photographs or casts) then the clinician's task is simplified. The effects of age-related changes on teeth and facial tissues, however, should not be forgotten. For example, the amount of central incisor tooth showing with the upper lip at rest in a teenager tends to be reduced with the passage of time. In addition, the dentist (and technician) should take into account other dentally related changes, such as physiological wear of teeth and age-related gingival recession (Fig. 4.26). Photographic features and/or peculiarities of mandibular anterior teeth and posterior teeth may also be determined. This photograph, however, must be usable; particularly useful are photographs of a patient that were taken when the subject was dentate or wore dentures they admired. The photographs should realistically show head-on facial views of the patient smiling, otherwise there

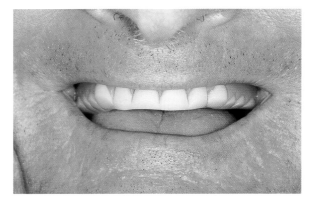

Fig. 4.26 Note obvious wear on the teeth and associated soft tissue changes.

will be no sign of the anterior teeth. Such views should enable the clinician to see and to measure carefully the ratio of the patient's horizontal intercanine distance and relate this to the interpupillary distance in the photograph. In the clinic the clinician may then measure the patient's interpupillary distance, and it should be possible to establish the horizontal width of the upper six anterior teeth. This was described earlier in the chapter. These guidelines are listed in Table 4.3.

In most cases, however, no adequate photographs or other pre-extraction records are available and the clinician has to decide on how best to select the teeth that will satisfy aesthetic and functional parameters. It is at this stage that guidelines relating to anterior tooth positioning may be used, and these guidelines are centred on the fact that the (six) maxillary anterior teeth should:

- Support the upper lip appropriately
- Occupy that area of the maxillary anterior arch bordered by the corners of the mouth
- Allow for individualisation where indicated, e.g. rotation, imbrication or spacing.

Many patients are satisfied with the appearance of their current dentures (or perhaps an earlier favoured denture) and there is much sense in repeating the prescription of moulds that are pleasing to the patient. To achieve this, the clinician should select the teeth on the basis of measurements and decisions made with the maxillary rim still in place, in order that functional and aesthetic parameters may be assessed. With the maxillary rim in place, the lip appropriately supported and the incisal point determined, the patient should be asked to smile. By marking the outline of the high smile line on the maxillary rim, the clinician is contributing to the development of one dimension to assist in the decision-making for tooth moulds (Fig. 4.27).

Two other important points to determine are the positions of the canine tips on the ACB. Earlier reference has been made to the use of pre-extraction records. Where these are not available, some authorities advocate using the position of the corners of the mouth, at rest, to determine the location of the canine points. Another method, used by the authors, is to ask the patient to smile

Table 4.4 List of factors influencing selection of posterior tooth form

Type of tooth	Occlusal factors	Stability factors	Aesthetic factors
Teeth with cusps	Balanced occlusion. Possible, but may require grinding to prevent slide from RCP to ICP. Balanced articulation. Cusps are required to obtain a truly balanced occlusion, but technician's skills and time are implicit, as is sound registration technique.	If no slide present, stability possible. Can be problematic with flat lower ridges and in implant-borne cases.	Tend to look better as they appear natural, as long as teeth of appropriate length are selected.
Teeth without cusps	Balanced occlusion. Possible and these teeth generally take less laboratory time to set up. Balanced articulation. A truly balanced articulation is not possible with these teeth.	Absence of cusps in the upper posterior teeth means balanced articulation is not possible.	Have a worn (attrited) appearance
Hybrid teeth	Balanced occlusion. Possible, some grinding may be necessary. Balanced articulation. Possible if concepts such as lingualised occlusion are used, i.e. the maxillary palatal cusps are intended to maintain contact with their antagonists	The presence of cusps, even modified cusps, can facilitate balanced articulation with reduced chance of cuspal locking	Can look natural

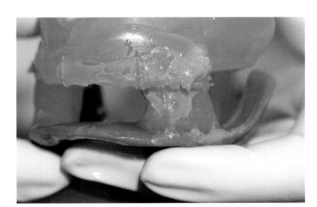

Fig. 4.27 The high smile line is indicated on the maxillary rim.

and to extend a line from the inner canthus of the eye via the lateral border of the alar cartilage and extend that on to the upper rim. This may be done with use of dental floss (see Fig. 4.9). This equates, in a high proportion of cases, to the position of the tip of the maxillary canine teeth.

The arc measured between the canine points on the ACB – the length of the 'aesthetic anterior arc' – can be read off. This reading is the second critical dimension required to prescribe tooth moulds (Fig. 4.28).

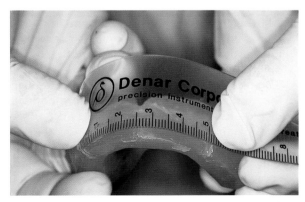

Fig. 4.28 The dimension of the anterior arch of the maxillary teeth is measured from distal of one canine to the other.

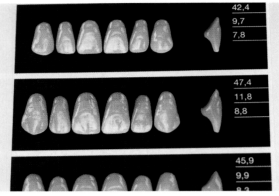

Fig. 4.29 Tooth mould charts indicating dimension of teeth.

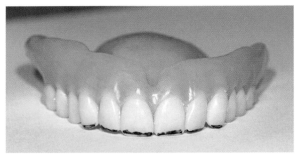

Fig. 4.30 The translucent tips of the central incisors have been blacked out to simulate wear in an older patient. The height of the blacked-out area should be subtracted from the height of the tooth indicated on the chart to achieve the desired height.

Prior to scrutinising mould charts, however, it is critically important that the clinician determines how the patient desires the tooth arrangement to look. If the patient wishes for spacing, then clearly that would require that narrower teeth be used to accommodate spacing in the aesthetic anterior arc. The converse is true where imbrication or crowding is desired. The importance of the two measurements is apparent when one examines most tooth mould charts. Figure 4.29 illustrates typical mould charts, in which dimensions are illustrated.

Three dimensions are given per mould:

- The combined widths of all six anterior teeth, i.e. from distal of canine to distal of the contralateral canine (in millimetres). NB: This is approximately the circumference of the upper rim from one canine point to the other <u>plus</u> 8–10 mm
- The height of the central incisors from the incisal edge to the highest point on the labial face of the tooth corresponding to the highest point of the crown (in mm)
- The width of the central incisors. Although the third value is of use in the prescription of removable partial dentures, we do not see any obvious value in the determination of tooth moulds for replacement complete dentures other than ensuring that replicated moulds are copied faithfully.

Armed with these two principal measurements, which may be read off the record rim, the clinician should be able to select from those moulds that lie within 1 mm of the selected intercanine distance. Similarly, an awareness of the dental changes with ageing is required when the height of the central incisors is being considered. The distance measured from the record rim is from the incisal tip to the high smile line. Most prosthodontic textbooks recommend that the highest point on the labial aspect of the crown lies 1 mm above this; clearly, for middle-aged and older patients modification of the central incisors will be required (i.e. remove the translucent tip of the incisal edge) to reflect the age of the patient (Fig. 4.30).

This will mean that the clinician, in order to customise the anterior teeth to reflect the age of the patient, will usually select longer central incisors than would be expected, to permit incisal grinding. On the other hand, some patients may not show much of their teeth when they smile. This may be a cultivated habit, for sociopsychological reasons, a consequence of tooth wear and a long upper lip, or perhaps simply a feature peculiar to these patients. This may be clear from a (good-quality) photograph of the patient smiling. It may also be apparent at the time of preparation of the ACB.

The clinician is, at all times, advised to consult the patient regarding his/her wishes and expectations on tooth selection, to help avoid – or at worst to minimise – any potential problems of acceptance of the replacement denture at a later date.

Clinical experience, however, indicates that even when these two measurements are followed, other factors are brought into play to finalise anterior tooth selection. Williams (1914) suggested that the frontal appearance of the face from the (normal) hairline to the chin could be used as a guideline to the inverse shape of the central incisor. Some tooth manufacturers, in an attempt to assist clinicians to select appropriate tooth moulds, suggest that the labial shape of the anterior tooth reflects the shape of the (edentulous) maxillary arch. Neither of these has any scientific credibility; indeed, the latter takes no account of trauma or unusual postextraction changes.

We recommend that clinicians should assess the facial profile in a three-dimensional way. This involves incorporating frontal and lateral views plus that taken from behind the patient looking down the face, to determine an overall view of the dentofacial profile. Patients from each of the skeletal classifications may be identified and this can help the clinician select a tooth mould which is in accordance with the profile of the appropriately supported lip on the basis of clinical experience of facial forms.

Selection of mandibular anterior teeth

As has already been mentioned, pre-extraction records may be used to facilitate appropriate tooth selection and, indeed, creation of the anterior form of the trial dentures. When these are not available, referral may be made to manufacturers' mould charts to equate the lower anterior teeth to the selected upper anterior teeth, or the practitioner may opt to create a functionally generated profile of the mandibular denture space (sometimes called the neutral-zone impression technique; Grant and Johnson 1992), identify the position of the lower canines (via the angle of the mouth), and then measure the canine–canine distance. As tooth moulds for mandibular anterior teeth have the equivalent three measurements to maxillary anterior teeth, the clinician may choose which mould is appropriate for each patient, taking age, facial form and patient perceptions into account.

Selection of posterior teeth types and moulds

It is probably accurate to state that this portion of the prescription form is least considered by clinicians, the choice of posteriors being often made by technicians who tend not to have seen the patient (McCord et al. 1992). This is a remarkable state of affairs when one considers that complete dentures are supposedly prescribed primarily to restore function and secondarily to restore facial appearance. As this book is intended for senior students and recent graduates, not specialists in prosthodontics, there will be no discussion on the geometry of occlusion and readers are referred to standard prosthodontic textbooks. It is pertinent, however, to discuss, albeit briefly, types of posterior teeth.

According to (Lang 1996), posterior tooth moulds are of four types:

- Anatomic
- Non-anatomic
- Zero-degree teeth
- Cuspless teeth.

According to the *Glossary of Prosthodontic Terms*, the following definitions apply to each type:

- **Anatomic**: teeth that have cuspal inclinations greater than 0° and tend to replicate occlusal anatomy. Such teeth may have cuspal angles set to 20°, 30°, 33° or 45°
- **Non-anatomic**: teeth designed in accordance with mechanical principles rather than from the anatomic standpoint
- **Zero-degree**: posterior teeth which have 0° cuspal angles
- **Cuspless**: teeth designed without cuspal prominence on the occlusal surface, i.e. inverted cusp teeth.

We would suggest, in the interests of clarity, that three types of posterior tooth form be considered, namely teeth with cusps, teeth without cusps, and teeth that exhibit both characteristics (hybrid moulds). The latter typically have maxillary teeth with cuspal angles of 20° with modified buccal cusps and mandibular non-anatomic teeth which have been rendered essentially cuspless.

The decision the clinician has to make should be determined according to the needs of the patient. In essence, three factors have to be considered, namely:

- Occlusal factors
- Stability factors
- Aesthetic factors.

Occlusal factors

If the patient only performs vertical mandibular movements then it is possible that cuspless teeth will suffice. If, however, the patient performs ruminatory mandibular movements (watch the patient eat a biscuit or a piece of carrot) then teeth with cusps will be required for balanced articulation (and thus stable dentures). Examination of current dentures may assist in the diagnosis. For example, if the dentures have occlusal surfaces which are evenly worn (i.e. flat), this is usually suggestive of vertical (chopping) mandibular movements, whereas much greater wear of the maxillary buccal cusps especially is suggestive of ruminatory mandibular movements (Fig. 4.31).

Stability factors

In addition to stability engendered out of muscle balance and occlusal balance in all border positions, cusps that tend to lock or cause tripping can worsen the stability of dentures. This is

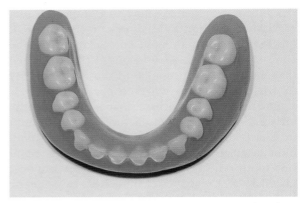

Fig. 4.32 Obvious undercuts present on the lingual surfaces of the mandibular molar teeth would result in instability.

particularly pronounced in flat, atrophic mandibular ridges. Some schools of thought automatically prescribe cuspless teeth in such cases; clearly, if balanced articulation is required the use of cuspless teeth is illogical. Another factor to consider is the width of the posterior teeth. If the posterior teeth are too broad they could present to the tongue what amounts to lingual undercuts, and the presence of these could lead to a major cause of instability (Fig. 4.32). The factors influencing the selection of posterior tooth form are listed in Table 4.4.

Thought should also be given to the number of posterior teeth. There are few clinical situations where there is sufficient mesiodistal length to incorporate two molars and two premolars without compromising stability (see Appendix 2); common options are to drop off either one premolar or one molar.

Aesthetic factors

This is something that can only be determined by the patient and is a good example of the value of informed consent: the patient should be informed of the options and allowed to decide on the appearance of posterior as well as anterior teeth.

Selection of colour and shade of teeth

As this book is intended to cover the broad principles of complete denture prosthodontics, no

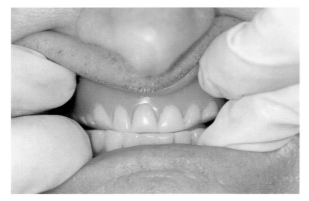

Fig. 4.31 Examination of the occlusal surfaces indicates clearly that the patient uses lateral excursions.

attempt will be made to detail the fundamentals of colour schemes. Although great care is often taken by dental practitioners over the selection of teeth of appropriate colours and shades for, for example, six anterior crowns, conventional wisdom would suggest that this is not the case where the selection of teeth for complete dentures is concerned.

Nevertheless, practitioners should take into account four qualities when selecting denture teeth. These are:

- **Hue**: This is a specific colour resulting from light of a particular wavelength acting on the retina. The hue is an indication of a specific colour, e.g. blue, green, reddish yellow. Some authorities suggest that the hue of teeth should harmonise with the hue of the patient's face/natural hair. Others, however, quote studies that cast doubt on this philosophy.
- **Chroma (saturation)**: This represents the amount of saturation of colour per unit area, for example one tooth may appear more yellow than another. The hue of both teeth could be equal, yet one could contain a higher saturation of a colour than the other.
- **Value (brilliance)**: This equates to the lightness or darkness of a tooth. Variations in brilliance are affected by dilution of the colour (i.e. the hue) by black or white. It is the ratio of white or black to the natural hue that determines the lightness or darkness of teeth.
- **Translucency**: This property enables light to pass through a body without giving any distinguishing image.

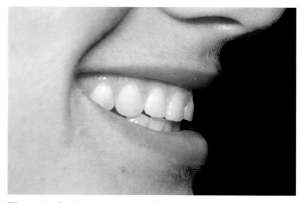

Fig. 4.33 In these natural teeth the canine is half a shade darker than the patient's incisor teeth.

The careful selection of colours and shades of teeth therefore verges on artistic interpretation. The patient may have very strong views about the shade of their replacement dentures, and therefore appropriate care in the selection of shades should be taken by the dental team (Landa 1988). Digital photography is a good way of enabling the technician to see the requirements of the patient if direct vision is not feasible. Shade selection may also be varied, for example there is often justification in having canine teeth slightly darker than incisors (Fig. 4.33).

When all of these details have been recorded on the laboratory (prescription) card, the rims may be dispatched to the laboratory for the trial dentures to be made, following routine infection control procedures.

REFERENCES

Academy of Prosthodontics. Glossary of prosthodontic terms. J Prosthet Dent 1999; 81: 1–142

Barsby MJ, Hellyer RP, Schwarz WD. The qualitative assessment of complete dentures produced by commercial dental laboratories. Br Dent J 1995; 179: 51–57

Basker RM, Ogden AR, Ralph JP. Complete denture prescription – an audit of performance. Br Dent J 1993; 174: 278–284

Brunton PA, McCord JF. An analysis of nasolabial angles and their relevance to tooth position in the edentulous patient. Eur J Prosthodont Rest Dent 1993; 2:53–56

Cabot LB. Using articulators to enhance clinical practice. Br Dent J 1997; 184: 272–276

Gonzalez JB. Preventing and treating abused tissue. In: Winkler S (ed). Essentials of complete prosthodontics, 2nd edn. St Louis: Mosby, 1988; 81–87

Grant AA, Heath JR, McCord JF. Complete prosthodontics: problems, diagnosis and management. London: Mosby Wolfe, 1994; 52–53

Grant AA, Johnson W. Introduction to removable denture prosthodontics, 2nd edn. Edinburgh: Churchill Livingstone, 1992

Landa LS. Anterior tooth selection and guidelines for complete denture aesthetics. In: Winkler S (ed). Essentials of complete denture prosthodontics, 2nd edn. St. Louis: Mosby, 1988; 202–221

Lang BR. Complete denture occlusion. Dent Clin North Am 1996; 40: 85–101

McCord JF, Firestone H, Grant AA. Phonetic determinants of tooth placement in complete dentures. Quint Int 1994; 25: 341–345

McCord JF, Grant AA, Quayle AA. Treatment options for the edentulous mandible. Eur J Prosthodontics Rest Dent 1992; 1: 19–23

McCord JF, Grant AA. Complete denture prosthetics. London: BDJ Books 2000

Morris HF. Recording bases and occlusal rims in essentials of complete denture prosthodontics. In: Winkler S (ed). Complete denture prosthodontics, 2nd edn. St Louis: Mosby, 1988; 123–136

Watt DM, MacGregor AR. Designing complete dentures, 2nd edn. Bristol: Wright, 1986; 2–31

Williams JL. A new classification of human tooth forms with special reference to a new system of artificial teeth. Dent Cosmos 1914; 56: 627–628

Zarb GA, Bolender CL, Hickey JL, Carlsson GE. Boucher's prosthodontic treatment of edentulous patients, 10th edn. St Louis: Mosby, 1990

5 Trial visits and insertion

The prescription, delivery and, indeed, success of complete denture treatment depends on the often imperceptible interaction of skills of clinicians (plus the dental nurses), the dental technician and, most important of all, the patient. The clinician, the team and the patient will already have established the needs and expectations of the patient, and this aspect has already been emphasised. Good communication should already have been practised between the dentist and the technician over the quality of casts and record rims.

The previous chapter outlined the registration visit, and the result of this is a three-dimensional prescription, appropriate for each patient, on which the denture teeth will be placed. Although the technical aspects of the try-in and processing stages are outlined in general in Chapter 7, it is essential that there be efficient communication between the technician and the clinical team if the next stage is to result in the creation of a set-up that satisfies the aesthetic and functional needs of the patient.

As with the other clinical stages, it should be a sine qua non that appropriate infection control procedures are practised.

The trial denture visits(s) are often seen as clinically easier (especially by students), but we would recommend that, in order to ensure that the appropriate result is achieved, the trial denture stage is practised meaningfully. In most instances, the trial dentures are delivered with the anterior teeth and posterior teeth in place and the wax bases contoured; if the appearance is perceived to be satisfactory to the patient and the dentist, and if the occlusion (generally only balanced occlusion in RCP) is perceived to be acceptable, then the denture is returned to the technician for processing. If, however, any changes are required to the arrangement of the teeth (either for aesthetic or functional reasons) then the technician is required to effect these changes and arrange for another trial visit.

Many clinicians feel less than comfortable about effecting these changes, and for this reason we recommend that two trial visits are arranged. The first is termed the aesthetic trial insertion.

In this visit, the trial dentures comprise the anterior teeth only in the maxillary and mandibular trial dentures, and the posterior segments comprise wax rims (Fig. 5.1). The clinician's task is simplified here, as there are five aspects to verify:

- That the anterior teeth have been selected appropriately, that the patient is content with the moulds selected and, further, that the arrangement of the teeth is to the liking of the patient. If the tooth moulds are incorrect, this may be easily modified by further discussion

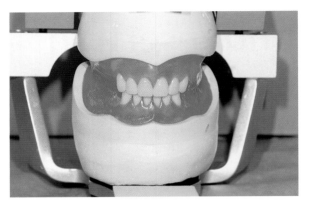

Fig. 5.1 Aesthetic (anterior) trial dentures.

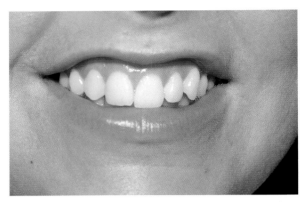

Fig. 5.3 The maxillary teeth conform to the smile line of the lower lip (note 1|1 represents incisal plane).

with the patient (the other three tasks may still be practised and the second trial visit may proceed as normal). If, however, the positioning or arrangement of the teeth requires to be altered, then the clinician can do this with relative ease at the chairside, as only six – or at worst 12 – anterior teeth need to be adjusted. If the teeth require to be raised (e.g. the maxillary anterior teeth are perceived to be too long) then the clinician may either raise them or indicate on the teeth the level desired (using a sharp wax pencil or felt-tipped pen; Fig. 5.2) so that the technician can adjust them. A good tip is to view the patient from the side and ask him/her to smile – the lower lip should lie parallel to the tips of the teeth of the maxillary

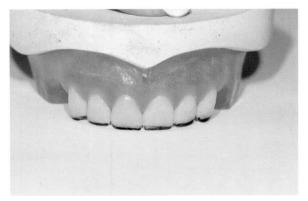

Fig. 5.2 A black felt-tipped pen has been used to indicate the desired incisal level of the maxillary anterior teeth.

denture (Fig. 5.3). NB: If the maxillary teeth are to be raised and the mandibular teeth to be kept at the same level (or *vice versa*) then the OVD needs to be lowered accordingly, and this needs to be communicated to the technician.

- That the retruded contact position (RCP) is acceptable. In simple terms this means that the wax rims representing the posterior occlusal segments contact evenly on both sides and along their lengths. If not, then this should be rectified by adding/removing wax accordingly. This is a relatively straightforward task for all clinicians to do.
- That the freeway space (FWS) determined is appropriate. This may be measured indirectly via an instrument such as the Willis bite gauge or similar, and related to that previously determined (see above). If an error has occurred, then the OVD may be increased or reduced as above.
- That speech is not impaired. This may partly be assessed in the verification of the FWS for sibilant sounds (ask the patient to say 'street', or count from 60 to 70; if prolonged 'S' sounds are detected this tends to indicate that the closest speaking distance is compromised, and the OVD should be reduced appropriately. Another useful tip here is to check labiodental sounds (e.g. 'f' or 'v'); in general, for English-speaking patients the tip of the maxillary central incisor teeth contacts the vermilion border of the lower lip.

- That the waxwork (gingival matrix) surrounding the teeth is appropriate and that it is acceptable to the patient. For example, some patients prefer to have the gingival matrix stippled, whereas others do not. Further details on waxing-up are presented in Chapter 7.

If the above checks are deemed to be acceptable, then the aesthetic trial dentures may be returned to the technician for conversion into the definitive trial dentures, ready for the second trial visit. This is termed the definitive trial insertion.

In this visit, the following six aspects have to be assessed/verified by the clinician:

- That the arrangement of the teeth meets with the agreement of the patient (and the clinician). We recommend that the patient be given some time to wear the trial dentures in the surgery, to enable them to become familiar with the feel of them before examining them in a mirror. It may also be useful for a friend/relative of the patient to be present (if the patient consents) to let them see what is being prescribed. Consent to proceed may then be recorded and verified if a 'witness' is present. Again, some personalisation of the dentures may be required. This may take the form of minor alteration to the arrangement of the teeth, or it may be a cosmetic inclusion in the denture, e.g. a gold inlay (Fig. 5.4) or spacing (Fig. 5.5). Another check concerns the placement of the mandibular posterior teeth over the residual ridge in the

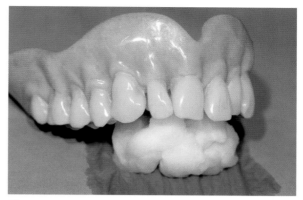

Fig. 5.5 Spacing has been incorporated. (NB: The clinician and the patient must decide whether the space is to be left 'as is' or filled with translucent acrylic – the latter is indicated where the space is minimal.)

interests of (mandibular) denture stability. This may be done by placing a wax knife on that portion of the impression surface corresponding to the residual ridge and then comparing that to the position of the central fossae of the posterior teeth (Fig. 5.6). Aberrant positioning should result in the trial denture being returned to the technician for appropriate placement of the teeth.

- That RCP is acceptable. This should be as per the previous visit. Failure to obtain a reproducible RCP may indicate that occlusal pivots are required; if this clinical option is

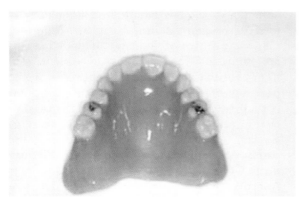

Fig. 5.4 Gold inlays have been added to the maxillary premolar teeth.

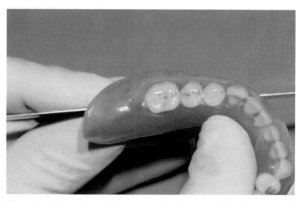

Fig. 5.6 A useful guide to verify that, in the interests of stability, the central fossae of the mandibular posterior teeth are positioned over the residual ridge.

not to be employed, then the clinician should re-register the RCP by removing the posterior teeth (e.g. of the maxillary trial denture) and re-registering the RCP. If this situation occurs, then the clinician should ask why an error has resulted and seek to eliminate clinical errors. Some patients, however, through no fault of their own, are unable to provide a reproducible RCP and, as has been mentioned above, assistance in the form of occlusal pivots may be worthy of consideration (see Case Study 2).

- That the FWS is appropriate. This should have been verified at the aesthetic trial insertion stage.
- That balanced articulation, if required, is present. This can only be partly assessed, as the teeth are held in place by wax and are not therefore able to withstand undue occlusal contacts. For that reason, if balanced articulation is required the clinician should stabilise the mandibular denture by placing his/her fingers on the wax flanges and requesting the patient to move from RCP into lateral and protrusive excursions (Fig. 5.7). Locking or tripping of the dentures during these excursions should be noted and the interferences marked. The clinician may remove the interferences (see below) or request that the technician do so prior to processing.
- That speech is not constrained. Again, this should have been checked at the aesthetic trial insertion stage.

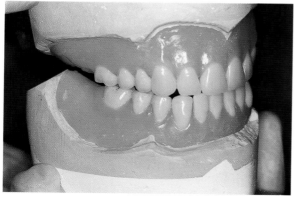

Fig. 5.7 The dentures have been moved into right lateral occlusion – the balancing points on the right are in contact.

- That the gingival matrix around anterior and posterior teeth conforms to prosthodontic norms appropriate for the patient. Included in this stage is the assessment of the wax periphery/extension. If the trial denture is overextended then the processed denture will be overextended. The clinician should therefore ensure that the periphery does not interfere with action of the cheeks, lips or tongue. This will be covered in greater detail in the section on insertion of processed dentures.

If these checks highlight errors, then a further trial insertion visit is indicated. If they prove that the trial dentures are acceptable then the clinician should verify that any further customisation is agreed and the information be conveyed to the technician.

Additional aspects to be conveyed to the technician are:

- **Type of base**. The usual base is made of poly (methyl) methacrylate (PMMA). The PMMA may be 'conventional' or strengthened by copolymers or other strengthening agents, e.g. fibres of carbon or other polymers. Sometimes patients prefer to have a metal base. This should ideally have been determined at the initial visit. Readers are reminded that if a metal base, e.g. cobalt–chromium, is prescribed then the postdam area should be so designed as to enable rebasing at a later date. If the patient has an allergy to PMMA, then an alternative base should be requested, e.g. polycarbonate, although only a few laboratories are equipped to offer this material.
- **Characteristics of the base**. Included in this are ethnic hues and perhaps translucent resin if it is felt that any spacing might result in the trapping of food (Fig. 5.8). Another option is that the patient's mandibular ridge is sufficiently atrophic to merit the prescription of a resilient lining (Fig. 5.9); equally, where patients have been prescribed resilient linings in previous dentures, they may prefer to have resilient linings!
- As was mentioned previously, the patient may request that a **restoration or a cosmetic feature** be incorporated in their denture (see Fig. 5.4). These features may not significantly

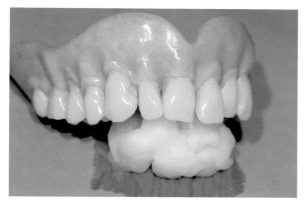

Fig. 5.8 Transparent resin imparts a semblance of spacing.

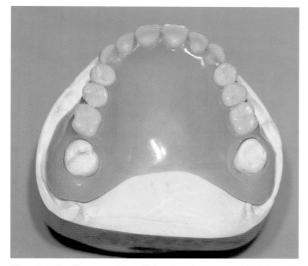

Fig. 5.9 A silicone rubber lining has been provided for this denture.

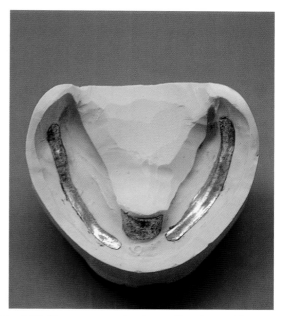

Fig. 5.10 The master cast has been relieved to avoid pressure over the patient's mobile mandibular ridge.

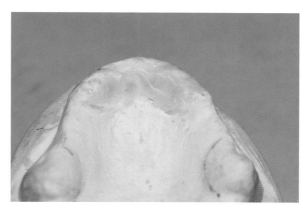

Fig. 5.11 Plaster has been added to the inter-rugal areas to reduce the potential for irritation caused by movement of the maxillary denture over/in these areas.

influence the retention, stability or function of the dentures, but they might significantly influence their acceptance by the patient.

- **Areas of relief that may be desired on the master cast prior to processing**. This may be indicated where there is overtly displaceable tissue (Fig. 5.10), or where the palatal rugae are deeply fissured (Fig. 5.11).
- **Provision of rugae where appropriate**. This feature is not commonly provided, but the authors commonly recommend it when, in rare cases, mandibular complete dentures are not

provided. In this instance the rugae may usefully provide a means of enhancing trituration of food by the tongue.

INSERTION STAGE

In the previous section we highlighted the benefits of approaching trial insertion in two stages/visits.

63

After a successful outcome, the dentures are processed and 'customised' if this is felt necessary. Proficiency in the trial insertion stage should mean that few clinical problems should be encountered at the insertion stage. Nevertheless, this stage should be performed in two temporal sections.

Assessment prior to the delivery of the dentures to the patient

Before the dentures are inserted into the patient's mouth, the clinician should carefully examine their three surfaces, namely the impression or 'fitting' surface of each denture, the polished surfaces of each denture, and the occlusal surfaces of each denture.

Impression surfaces

The surfaces should be examined independently and sharp or rough areas removed. These may be identified by palpation of those areas of the denture base that will be in close contact with the denture-bearing tissues or via teased cotton wool (Fig. 5.12). An acrylic bur may then be used to smooth the surface. As the processed dentures should be returned on the master casts or replicas of them, the clinician should ensure that the dentures do not rock on the casts, as this might indicate potential instability in the inserted dentures. This is most commonly assessed by

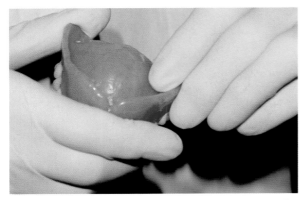

Fig. 5.12 Sharp areas on the impression surface may be palpated even with a gloved finger.

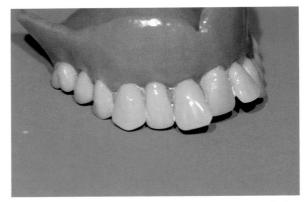

Fig. 5.13 Poor technique has resulted in acrylic resin flashes covering the denture teeth.

pressing with the index fingers on the premolar teeth, first on one side and then the other.

Polished surfaces

These surfaces should be closely examined to ensure that the gingival matrix has been proficiently finished. Typical points to look out for are flashes of pink extending on to the teeth (Fig. 5.13). This indicates a less than ideal technical procedure and the dentures should be returned to the technician for correction. Equally, as was indicated in Chapter 3, the peripheral roll should have been preserved on the master cast and the periphery should conform to this if proficient, non-patient-determined retention is to be achieved.

Occlusal surfaces

Three areas are important here. First, the occlusal and incisal surfaces should be assessed to ensure that no roughened areas or chipped surfaces are present. The second relates to the placement of the mandibular posterior teeth over the residual ridge in the interests of (mandibular) denture stability. This was covered in the section on trial insertion (Fig. 5.6).

The third area to examine is the occlusion. The processed dentures should ideally be returned from the laboratory on the master casts, and either on an articulator or on mounting plates such that the dentist may assess the occlusion of the dentures *in vitro*. A necessary attribute of all dentures is that there should be balanced occlusion in RCP – this is easily checked on the articulator by ensuring that the posterior teeth touch uniformly and evenly. If balanced articulation was requested, then this should be demonstrable on the articulator; this means that there is even sliding contact of the supporting cusps of the posterior teeth from RCP to right and left lateral and protrusive excursions. Equally, the incisor teeth should not cause tripping of the mandibular denture in protrusion.

When these assessments have been performed, the dentures should be placed in an appropriate infection control medium before being prepared for the second phase of predelivery inspection.

Assessment of the dentures in the patient

If the initial assessment is favourable, the clinician may then proceed with an *in vivo* assessment of the processed dentures. There are a variety of ways in which this may be carried out, but we recommend that it be done in three stages.

Assessment of the maxillary denture

Having ensured that there are no blemishes on the impression surface (that might induce support problems), the maxillary denture may be inserted. Pain on insertion may indicate the presence of undercuts. These may be located via pressure-indicating paste and relieved (Fig. 5.14). Not all undercuts, however require to be relieved: indeed some may well be used to optimise retention (Fig.5.15).

The stability of the denture may be assessed by digital pressure on the premolar teeth to ensure that no rocking occurs. If it does, this generally indicates a discrepancy between the denture-bearing tissues and the impression surface of the denture – an impression for a rebase is generally indicated. Another aspect of stability of the maxillary denture is the periphery. Placing the index finger of the left hand on the middle of the palate, tug gently on the right cheek; if

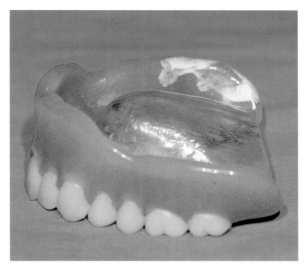

Fig. 5.14 Pressure-indicating paste has been removed from the denture at an undercut area of the tuberosity.

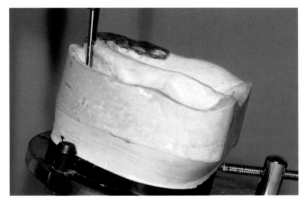

Fig. 5.15 The undercut inherent in the anterior ridge may be utilised by having an upwards and backwards path of insertion – the path of insertion is indicated on the master cast.

displacement/movement of the denture occurs, the periphery is overextended. Again, pressure-indicating paste is a useful clinical tool to locate the area of overextension. The excess may be removed with an acrylic bur and the process repeated to ensure that the (right) buccal periphery of the denture is not overextended. A similar procedure may then be used to ensure that the left periphery is not overextended.

Problems of support may be further tested by standing behind the patient and gently pressing the denture into the denture-bearing tissues by the (gloved) fingertips of the operator. Areas of discomfort may be identified with pressure-relief paste and subsequently relieved.

Overextension of the labial flange may be assessed by asking the patient to purse his/her lips; if the denture drops, then the periphery should be reduced after the area of excess has been identified via the use of impression paste.

NB: The roughened areas of the periphery arising out of removal of overextension should be polished before delivering the dentures definitively.

Assessment of the mandibular denture

Essentially the same procedures advocated for the maxillary denture should be followed for the mandibular denture. The principal difference concerns the assessment of the extension of the lingual aspect of the mandibular denture. Placing the index fingers on the buccal flanges of the denture, the operator should ask the patient to touch the tip of the upper lip with the tongue. If the denture is displaced, the lingual periphery is overextended; using pressure-indicating paste on first the left then the right peripheries will identify areas of overextension (Fig. 5.16), which may then be relieved. In contrast, however, if the patient can protrude his/her tongue fully without displacing the denture, then the denture is underextended lingually and serious consideration should be given to recording an impression for

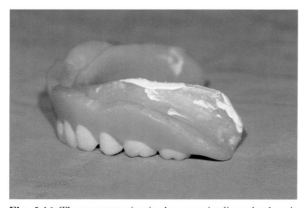

Fig. 5.16 The overextension in the posterior lingual sulcus is indicated by the removal of pressure-indicating paste.

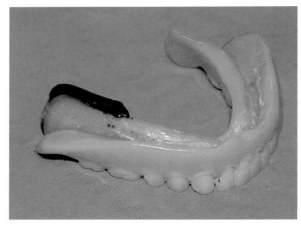

Fig. 5.17 Greenstick tracing compound has been moulded to form an appropriate lingual extension prior to relining the denture. This should improve resistance to lateral movement of the denture.

relining of the mandibular denture, after the extension has been appropriately moulded using, for example, greenstick tracing compound (Fig. 5.17).

Assessment of occlusion

This requires that the maxillary and mandibular dentures be inserted; to avoid any unnecessary discomfort to the patient, it is recommended that the mandibular denture is inserted first, followed by the maxillary denture. This is because the appropriately extended maxillary denture will support the lips and cheeks, and subsequent insertion of the mandibular denture might stretch the tender tissues at the angles of the mouth.

The first aspect to assess is that balanced occlusion occurs in RCP. Articulating paper may be used to ensure that there are even contacts between the supporting cusps of the maxillary premolar and molar teeth (palatal cusps) and the central fossae/marginal ridges of the mandibular premolar and molar teeth. The same rationale is expected for the supporting cusps of the mandibular posterior teeth (the buccal cusps) and the central fossae/marginal ridges of the posterior maxillary teeth. Figure 5.18 illustrates an example of even contacts on the opposing maxillary/mandibular teeth. In this instance no remedial action is required. Figure 5.19, however, illustrates

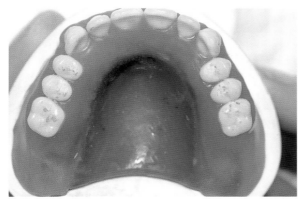

Fig. 5.18 Even bilateral contacts on the posterior teeth.

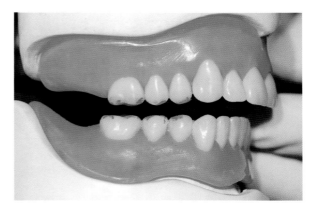

Fig. 5.20 The areas marked indicate where the buccal cusps of the posterior teeth need to be relieved to correct a protrusive slide.

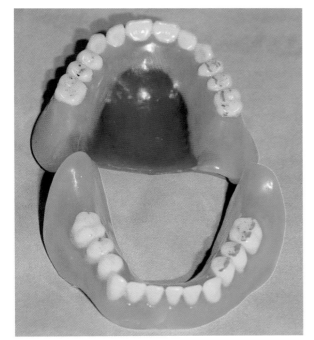

Fig. 5.19 Obvious contacts on maxillary central fossae and marginal ridges plus mandibular supporting cusps and marginal ridges.

an example where there is a heavy contact on the patient's right molar teeth. This should be rectified by easing the heavy contacts **in the central fossae and marginal ridges, not the supporting cusps**.

If there is a protrusive slide from RCP into ICP, amounting to a half cusp width, this may be remedied by identifying the premature contacts and easing the **mesial-facing** cusps of the maxillary buccal cusps and the **distal-facing** cusps of the mandibular buccal cusps (Fig. 5.20). Where the protrusive slide equates to more than a quarter of the cusp width, the occlusion should be reregistered and the posterior occlusion reset.

With respect to balanced articulation (and assuming that it is prescribed for the patient) the authors tend not to be overcritical of the assessment of lateral excursions at this visit, owing to the fact that some degree of displacement of tissues and some adjustment of the patient to the new dentures is likely to occur. For that reason, the assessment of excursive movements will be dealt with in Chapter 6.

INSTRUCTIONS TO THE PATIENT

It is good practice to provide written advice to patients with regard to:

- How to cope with new dentures
- When to attend for review
- How to look after the dentures
- Future maintenance of the dentures.

Many dental practitioners have booklets on the above: indeed, many booklets on denture care are provided by commercial companies. A simple leaflet informing patients how to cope with new dentures is illustrated in Figure 5.21.

UNIVERSITY DENTAL HOSPITAL, MANCHESTER

DEPARTMENT OF PROSTHETIC DENTISTRY

INSTRUCTIONS TO PATIENTS RECEIVING FULL DENTURES

A great deal of care and skill has been used in the production of the denture(s) which you have received. To enable you to learn to use the dentures as quickly as possible and get the greatest benefit from them you are asked to note the following advice:—

(1) Eating may be difficult at first. Cut your food into small pieces, and take your time chewing. Avoid tough and sticky foods over the learning period.

(2) Remove your dentures and clean them after each meal. A soft brush with soap and cold water are satisfactory for cleaning. Alternatively, a proprietary denture cleaner may be used, following the manufacturers' instructions.

(3) Remove your dentures at night and store in water to prevent them drying out and warping.

(4) Pain and soreness sometimes occur with new dentures. Adjustment may be required. If the pain is severe, leave the dentures out and arrange an appointment with your dentist as soon as possible. Wear the dentures the day you return to the dentist so that the sore area may be seen.

Never attempt to adjust the denture yourself.

a

Fig. 5.21 (a)

UNIT OF PROSTHODONTICS

CARE FOR YOUR DENTURES

- ## WHY IS IT IMPORTANT TO LOOK AFTER THEM?

    - **Prevent bad breath**
    - **Keep them looking good**
    - **Help your mouth to stay healthy**

- ## HOW SHOULD YOU LOOK AFTER THEM?

    Our recommendations for effective cleansing of plastic dentures are:-

    - Rinse denture after every meal.
    - Remove debris by brushing with a soft brush, soap and cold water.
    - Ensure this is done over a sink of water to avoid breakage should the denture fall.
    - Soak denture for 10 minutes each evening in Dentural or Milton solution.
    - Rinse thoroughly with cold water, then soak overnight in water in a closed container. (This is not always practical)

- ## SPECIAL SITUATIONS

    We recommend the following procedures to deal with specific instances

    Tartar on Dentures:

    Hard deposits (calculus) on dentures are difficult to remove.
    Acid based cleaners such as Denclen and Deepclean are most effective (*but not to be used for metal dentures*), if deposits persist see your dentist.

    Metal Based Dentures:

    Any dentures containing metal can be damaged by **ACID** cleansers such as Denclen, Deepclean etc.,
    If you buy a proprietary cleaner be sure it is **NOT ACID !!!** – (ACIDIC)

    It is safe to soak metal based dentures in effervescent cleansers such as Steradent or Boots Effervescent/Double Action for fifteen minutes. Alternatively soak in Dentural or Milton for ten minutes each evening.

    Soft Linings:

    These are prone to damage – **AVOID**
    - Hard brushes
    - Toothpaste and effervescent cleansers (Steradent, Boots Effervescent/Double Action)

- ## PLEASE REMEMBER

    - Always follow manufacturers' instructions when using proprietary cleansers
    - If you have any questions – please ask our staff
    - Have your mouth and dentures checked regularly by a professional. **TIG 80/99**

b

Fig. 5.21 (a) and (b) Patient information leaflets.

Many clinicians are of the opinion that delivery of replacement dentures is an end-process. Experienced clinicians recognise that this is not the case and that it is most unlikely that no future treatment will be required in the short term. What is certain, however, is that residual ridge resorption is continuous and irrevocable, and therefore the dentures will need to be relined/rebased or even replaced after 5 years or more. For some people this period may be shorter than 5 years. For that reason, it is important that the clinician is aware of his/her responsibilities for what is required for review and maintenance. This is the subject of Chapter 6.

6 Review and maintenance

REVIEW

The first review visit for a patient who has recently received dentures is seldom without difficulty. In the experience of the authors, a patient who presents without a problem is the exception rather than the rule. This chapter discusses common problems encountered at review and offers potential solutions in a systematic way.

Although every care may have been taken at previous visits, the inevitability of dealing with postinsertion problems necessitates this chapter. Common practice is for the first review appointment to be made one week after insertion of the dentures. This timing, however, would not appear to be based on any evidence. Unpublished data would appear to indicate that some problems are likely to occur after a period of three days. It would therefore seem sensible to review the patient after this period of time.

What is crucial is to establish that this visit is every bit as important as the other visits previously described and ought therefore to be conducted with care and attention.

The review visit may be made much less disappointing for the patient and dentist if, at the insertion stage, care is given to informing the patient what problems might be expected to arise afterwards. In this respect, if the patient is forewarned they are forearmed, and hopefully less disappointed about any discomfort or other problems that may arise.

Problems encountered at the review visit may be classified as follows, as in Chapter 2:

- Appearance
- Function
- Comfort
- Speech
- Psychological
- Other.

Appearance

Problems with appearance may occasionally arise at the delivery visit and are disappointing for all concerned. Problems tend to arise when communication has broken down, and may therefore usually be avoided if care has been taken in the previous visits to inform the patient fully of the scope and limitations of the treatment being undertaken. Careful management of the patient at the trial insertion visit normally overcomes most of the difficulties. However, one problem that may arise is where a relative or close companion dislikes the end result. This may be avoided by encouraging patients to bring a relative or trusted friend along with them during the try-in visit. When this is not feasible, the patient can be invited to take the try-in home with them for a longer assessment of the appearance by him/ herself and whoever else has an interest. It is often helpful in such cases to ask the patient to make a list of what they like or dislike to help achieve a more desirable end result.

Where the aesthetic problems relate to colour it is possible, in certain circumstances, to make changes to the denture. Where teeth are perceived as being too light, surfaces may be stained using proprietary staining kits. In the experience of the authors this may allow teeth to be darkened, although the staining is readily removed. However, where the shade selected is too dark, it is probably better to consider removal and resetting of replacement teeth.

If the patient expresses disappointment with tooth position, grinding the teeth may help resolve the problem, but removal of the teeth and a retry may be the only sensible option. At this stage, the modification of the polished surface must also be considered to establish whether this aspect of the denture affects patient satisfaction.

Function

With respect to function, the patient may report several difficulties.

Looseness of dentures

In all but a very few patients a loose mandibular denture should be expected, owing to the inherent problems of stability in an atrophic mandibular arch (McCord et al. 1992). Looseness of the mandibular denture may only be predictably reduced by the placement of dental implants to help increase retention. This has become more standard practice and should be considered during initial planning. Where conventional treatment is carried out, the patient should have been warned that some degree of 'looseness', particularly of the mandibular denture, is likely.

Without such counselling, the expectations of the patient may be higher than can be managed.

Patients may describe the term 'looseness' in different ways, such as:

- Rocking or shifting of the maxillary denture
- Falling of the mandibular denture
- Rising or lifting
- 'The dentures are too big', implying that the patient considers that they do not fit the residual ridge and are therefore loose
- The dentures are bulky and occupy too much space in the mouth.

It is therefore helpful to question the patient as to what is meant by their wording.

With respect to the maxillary denture the converse occurs, with retention problems being more the exception than the rule. If the impression procedures were performed correctly fewer difficulties are likely to arise, but when they do the following approach may serve to establish the cause(s). To help in the diagnosis of this complaint, the causes of looseness and their management will now be discussed.

Causes of lack of retention

There are numerous causes of apparently loose dentures, any or many of which may result in the above symptoms. Accurate diagnosis of the cause of looseness is therefore essential, otherwise the problem is unlikely to be overcome when modifying existing dentures or avoided when constructing new appliances. As the diagnosis is not always obvious, time is well spent listening to what patients say is wrong with their dentures. Their response to pertinent questions can be most helpful, alongside careful observation of the dentures inside and outside the mouth, of the lips, cheeks and tongue when static and in function, and of the denture-supporting tissues; and in palpation of both hard and soft tissues. Causes of loose dentures may be classified as follows:

- Decreased retentive forces
  - Lack of peripheral seal (Fig. 6.1)
  - Air beneath the impression surface
  - Xerostomia
  - Neuromuscular control.

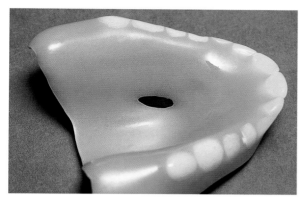

Fig. 6.1 The hole in this denture compromises the peripheral seal.

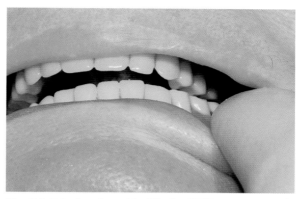

Fig. 6.3 It is clear from this slide that RCP was not properly recorded.

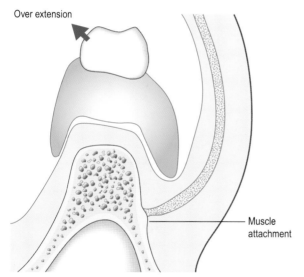

Over extension

Muscle attachment

Fig. 6.2 This slide illustrates how overextension of the denture can compromise stability by interfering with molar attachments.

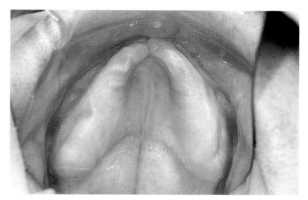

Fig. 6.4 This slide shows 'flabby ridges anteriorly', which represents absence of bone in the ridge.

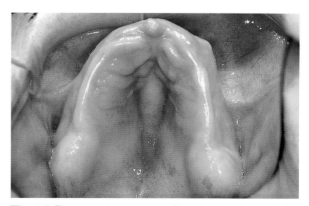

- Increased displacing forces
  - Denture border problems (e.g. overextension) (Fig. 6.2)
  - Occlusal problems (Fig. 6.3).
- Support problems
  - Lack of ridge (Fig. 6.4)
  - Bony prominence(s) (Fig. 6.5)
  - Non-resilient soft tissue (Fig. 6.6)
  - Pain-avoidance mechanisms.

Fig. 6.5 Bony prominences are evident in the palate and also on the patient's upper right maxillary canine area.

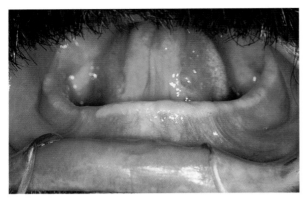

Fig. 6.6 The blanching represents areas of atrophic mucosa, and this would need to be relieved on the master cast.

For ease of reading, these causes, and their presentation and management are displayed in Tables 6.1 to 6.7.

OCCLUSAL ADJUSTMENT OF DENTURES

For all but the most minor occlusal errors the occlusal adjustment of dentures is most easily and best carried out in the dental laboratory. Minor occlusal adjustment may be carried out

clinically if the initial tooth contact during closure in the retruded contact position (RCP) may be visualised and is seen to be coincident with the intercuspal position of the denture and at the appropriate occlusal vertical dimension.

Where 'slides' occur during mandibular closure, accurate clinical identification of 'early' occlusal contacts is often extremely difficult. This is because marks may still result after the slide has occurred that may not be representative of what would result if the slide had not happened. 'True' markings in the RCP of the mandible (where a slide is present) are therefore best made by recording the RCP accurately, mounting the maxillary denture on an articulator via a facebow transfer, and relating the mandibular cast to the maxillary cast using an accurate interocclusal record. The only difference from this procedure and that described in a previous chapter is that the RCP is recorded where the denture teeth are present rather than via wax rims. The fact that the dentures should be more retentive after having been processed makes recording RCP at this stage much easier. Wax may be placed over the occlusal aspects of the denture teeth of the mandibular denture and indents made into the wax on closure in RCP. Care must be made to ensure tooth

Table 6.1 Causes of loose dentures – decreased retentive forces – lack of seal

Cause	Presentation	Management
Border underextension in depth	On delivery When speaking When eating When opening wide After adjustment	For all problems of lack of seal, modification of the denture border depth and width with greenstick may improve the border seal to confirm the problem. Subsequent reline/rebase may be performed at the chairside if the modification is minor. For greater modification of the denture, relining or rebasing is better carried out in the dental laboratory
Border underextension in width	As above	
Posterior border of upper denture	As above	
Resorption of residual ridge	After some months of satisfactory wear	
Inelasticity of cheeks	On delivery When speaking When eating When opening wide After adjustment After some months of satisfactory wear	

Table 6.2 Causes of loose dentures – decreased retentive forces – air beneath impression surface

Cause	Presentation	Management
Undercut ridge	When eating After adjustment	Utilisation of undercut is advantageous to denture retention. A planned path of rotational insertion may enable undercut to be used without causing trauma to the soft tissues
Excessive relief chamber	As above	See below
Poor fit		
Poor impression	On delivery When eating	Check for any rocking or any gaps between the flanges and the tissues. A reline technique may be used to improve the adaptation of the denture to the tissues
Damaged cast	As above	
Warped denture	On delivery When eating After adjustment	
Over-adjustment	After adjustment	
Resorption of residual ridge	After some months of satisfactory wear	
Change in tissue fluid	On delivery When eating After some months of satisfactory wear Looseness following immediate/recent illness	

Table 6.3 Causes of loose dentures – decreased retentive forces – xerostomia

Cause	Presentation	Management
Xerostomia		
Lack of or diseases of salivary glands	On delivery When speaking When eating When opening wide After adjustment After some months of satisfactory wear	Consider whether the prescription of artificial saliva or a denture fixative may help retention
Irradiation of the head and neck	Looseness following immediate/recent illness	It is very unlikely that medication can be changed, but it is worth liaising with the general medical practitioner to see if alternative medication could be offered. This is more the case with antidepressants, as newer, more selective drugs have fewer side effects
Medications	As above As above	

contact has not occurred, as this may encourage some mandibular deviation. Should any areas of the wax appear thin, the procedure can be repeated until the clinician is satisfied that no deviation has occurred. A facebow transfer should be made and the dentures mounted on an articulator to allow occlusal analysis and subsequent adjustments to be carried out.

Table 6.4 Causes of loose dentures – decreased retentive forces – neuromuscular control

Cause	Presentation	Management
Neuromuscular control Shape incorrect	On delivery When speaking When eating After adjustment After some months of satisfactory wear	For all difficulties relating to control, it is the case that once they have been diagnosed, they are better managed. Problems of tooth position may relate to the mandibular molar teeth being placed too far lingually, thereby cramping the tongue. Removal of the lingual cusps may increase the tongue space. With the maxillary denture the teeth may be placed too far palatally, necessitating their removal and repositioning. A convex lingual polished surface may compromise denture stability and may be adjusted to be more divergent from the denture flange to the occlusal surface. Where there is an apparent improvement in retention with regard to the old dentures, but less patient satisfaction, a replica technique may be needed. The use of denture fixatives is recommended for ongoing problems of neuromuscular control
Motor neurone disorder	As above	
Change in shape relative to the old dentures	On delivery When speaking When eating After adjustment	
High occlusal plane on lower denture	When speaking When eating	
Patient does not appreciate the need for active control	When eating After adjustment	

Table 6.5 Causes of loose dentures – increased displacing forces – denture border problems

Cause	Presentation	Management
Denture border problems Overextension in depth	On delivery When speaking When eating When opening wide After adjustment	Overextension may be diagnosed by direct vision with manipulation of the soft tissues to identify the offending areas. Subsequent adjustment may then be carried out. Pressure-indicating creams may be helpful, but only if used locally
Overextension in width	As above	
Deep postdam on upper	As above	The patient may present with pain in the postdam area or ulceration/inflammation on examination in that area. The dam may be reduced, but caution should be exercised as decreased retention may also be the result of an inadequate seal

By way of a general guide, the following regimen may be used to make occlusal adjustments on the articulator:

1. **Errors in RCP**. In general, the reduction of certain cusp tips should be avoided. In particular, the mandibular buccal cusps and the maxillary palatal cusps should only be tampered with as a last resort, as they are required as centric 'stops' and also for balancing the occlusion on the non-working side in lateral excursions. In addition, it is considered helpful to attempt to adjust only one arch at a time, as this may help reduce the inadvertent result of overzealous reduction.

Thin articulating paper of a prescribed colour should be used for marking contacts made in RCP, which should be different

Table 6.6 Causes of loose dentures – increased displacing forces – occlusal problems

Cause	Presentation	Management
Occlusal problems		
Uneven initial contact	When eating After adjustment After some months of satisfactory wear	Problems relating to the occlusion may be considered either minor or major. Minor adjustments may be made at the chairside, but major problems are best addressed in the dental laboratory. More detailed description of occlusal adjustments is seen later in the main body of the text
Lack of occlusal balance in protrusive and lateral excursions	As above	
Lack of freedom in intercuspal position	When eating After some months of satisfactory wear	
Intercuspal and retruded contact positions not coincident	As above	
Excessive vertical overlap of teeth	On delivery When eating	
Last lower teeth too posteriorly placed	When eating	
Orientation of occlusal plane	When eating	

Table 6.7 Causes of loose dentures – support problems

Cause	Presentation	Management
Support problems		
Lack of ridge	On delivery When eating After some months of satisfactory wear	Consideration of the placement of dental implants with precision attachments
Bony prominence	As above	Relief over the region may be diagnosed with the use of relief creams and subsequently adjusted
Fibrous, displaceable ridge	On delivery When eating After adjustment After some months of satisfactory wear	Use of an impression technique as described in previous chapter (greenstick/compo or window technique)
Non-resilient soft tissue	As above	Use of an impression technique as described in previous chapter (admix of greenstick/compo)
Pain avoidance mechanisms	When eating After adjustment After some months of satisfactory wear After some months of satisfactory wear	Eliminate the cause of the pain

from the subsequent marking up of contacts made in excursive movements. Unwanted tooth contacts may be reduced by denture tooth adjustment as needed to gain bilateral, even contact. For details of the areas of teeth to be ground see Chapter 5.

2. **Errors in protrusive and lateral movements**. Errors in protrusive and lateral movements may be easily seen, if on these movements the denture/s are dislodged from the/their casts. The markings made in these excursions should be made in a different colour from that used in RCP to avoid the removal of any needed 'stops'. In this way, the denture teeth may be adjusted to achieve balanced occlusion. It is customary to consider the working and balancing sides independently, but the clinician should be mindful of the need to consider both. Working interferences are best dealt with using what is termed the 'BULL' rule, i.e. the palatal-facing surfaces of the **B**uccal **U**pper cusps and the buccal facing surfaces of the **L**ower **L**ingual

cusps. Balancing interferences may be identified and relieved by light grinding, taking care not to imperil centric stops.

Where, on mounting, or after occlusal adjustment, an acceptable occlusal relationship is not achieved, the denture teeth may need to be ground off and new teeth reset to the desired position.

COMFORT

It is almost inevitable that some discomfort will follow the delivery of dentures to a patient and in view of this it is wise to explain this to the patient well in advance. It is also considered good practice to establish, at the delivery visit, where potential problem areas are likely to be. Tables 6.8 to 6.13 serve as a template for the recognition and management of causes of discomfort.

SPEECH

Speech difficulties, fortunately, appear to be a relatively uncommon problem relating to denture

Table 6.8 Causes of discomfort related to the impression surface

Cause	Presentation	Management

Pressure areas due to:
    Faulty impression
    Damage to the working cast
    Warping of base during
    processing
    Immersing in too hot water
	On delivery
	When eating
	When swallowing
	As day progresses
	All the time
	After months of wear
		Initially, support problems may be recognised via digital pressure on the occlusal surfaces of the denture in situ. Pain on pressing the denture with the hands indicates a potential support/stability problem, e.g. fit. Use of pressure-indicating pastes (placed on the tissues and picked up on the denture) may help identify areas where further relief is required. Pain on biting may indicate an occlusal problem, which may be identified using articulating paper

Denture base not relieved in a region of undercut	On delivery When eating As day progresses All the time	Pain usually present on insertion and removal of dentures. Ulceration and erythematous areas may result. Again, place pressure-identifying paste on area affected, identify the appropriate area on the denture and relieve the denture accordingly
Pearls of acrylic or sharp ridges on the fitting surface of the denture	On delivery When eating When swallowing As day progresses All the time	Run thin wisps of cotton wool over the impression surface to identify area and then adjust with denture bur

Table 6.9 Causes of discomfort related to the impression surface

Cause	Presentation	Management
Lack of appropriate relief over tori, atrophic mucosa	On delivery When eating When swallowing As day progresses All the time	Examine the mouth for areas of atrophic mucosa and palpate with the finger. Adjust the denture in those areas identified as being problematic NB: This should have been identified and noted at first visit

Overextension of periphery
    Unrelieved frena or muscle attachments
    Pinching of tissue between denture base and tuberosity/retromolar pad
	When speaking
	When eating
	When opening wide
	When swallowing
	As day progresses
	After months of wear
		Manipulate the soft tissues with the denture in situ. Overextension present may cause the denture to be displaced and/or blanching of the area of overextension. Lack of relief for frena is usually accompanied by pain and ulceration

Mandibular denture overextended and pressing on mylohyoid ridge(s)	When eating When swallowing All the time	Manipulate the soft tissues with the denture in situ. Overextension present may cause the denture to be displaced and/or blanching of the tissues in the area of overextension. Lifting of the tongue may displace the denture. Reduce the overextension until the tongue may be protruded without the denture being displaced

Table 6.10 Causes of discomfort related to the impression surface

Cause	Presentation	Management
Atrophic mucosa/spiky ridge	On delivery When eating When swallowing As day progresses All the time After months of wear	Identify areas with pressure-indicating paste and adjust as required. Atrophic mucosa may preclude satisfactory denture-wearing and consideration may be given to enhancing the support for the denture by placement of dental implants
Postdam too deep	On delivery When speaking When eating When swallowing As day progresses All the time After months of wear	First check that the occlusal vertical dimension of occlusion is appropriate. If so, reduce the postdam depth but with caution, as excess reduction may compromise retention

Table 6.11 Causes of discomfort related to the polished surfaces

Cause	Presentation	Management
Maxillary denture constraining coronoid process	When speaking When eating When opening wide	Discomfort evident on opening and closing of the mandible or in lateral movements of the mandible during function. Use of pressure-indicating pastes may enable the offending area to be identified and adjusted

Table 6.12 Causes of discomfort related to the occlusal surfaces

Cause	Presentation	Management
Slide from retruded contact position to intercuspal position	Pain and/or ulceration lingual to the mandibular ridge anteriorly When eating When swallowing As day progresses	See earlier section on occlusal adjustment
Lack of incisal overjet	Pain and/or ulceration labial to the mandibular ridge anteriorly When speaking When eating When swallowing As day progresses	See earlier section on occlusal adjustment
Lack of appropriate freeway space	When eating When swallowing As day progresses	See earlier section on occlusal adjustment
Lack of occlusal contacts	When eating When swallowing As day progresses All the time	See earlier section on occlusal adjustment

Table 6.13 Discomfort related to other causes

Cause	Presentation	Management
Instability of dentures	On delivery When eating When swallowing As day progresses After months of wear	Examine all aspects of the denture for possible causes and rectify if possible Consider the placement of dental implants to improve stability if at all possible
Burning mouth syndrome	All the time After months of wear When dentures out	Consider a referral to a specialist in oral medicine
Xerostomia	On delivery When eating When swallowing All the time When dentures out	Use of artificial saliva Use of analgesic mouthrinse prior to eating ? Consider liaison with GP to change medication if possible
TMD	On delivery When eating When opening wide After months of wear	Check all aspects of the complete dentures are appropriate ? Soft diet, TENS, physiotherapy, analgesia or other medication

wearing. When they do arise, however, they can be very taxing for both the patient and the clinician. Tables 6.14 and 6.15 outline the possible problems of speech and their management.

PSYCHOLOGICAL

Underlying psychological problems may have an adverse effect on the successful wearing of

Table 6.14 Management of speech problems

Speech problem	Recognition	Management
Noise on eating/speaking	Excessive OVD Occulusal interferences Loose dentures	Remake dentures at reduced OVD Occlusal adjustment See previous chapter
General speech problems – initial – longer term		Reassurance See below
Sibilants, e.g. 's'	Ask the patient to count from 60 to 70. The maxillary and mandibular incisor teeth should be just out of contact. If in contact, selective grinding will be required. If severe, a reset may be advisable	See chapter on managing the vertical dimension of occlusion. Also, the palatal contours of the denture may be checked with the use of disclosing creams for excess contact. Lack of contact may be assessed using wax additions

Table 6.15 Management of speech problems (continued)

Speech problem	Recognition	Management
Bilabial sounds, e.g. 'p' and 'b'	Is the lip approximation easily attained? Incorrect incisal position	Check the OVD Remove the incisors and reset new ones in wax and reassess
Labiodental sounds, e.g. 'f' and 'v'	Does the vermilion border of the mandibular lip rest against the incisal edges of the upper teeth? On swallowing, does the mandibular lip overlap the labial surface of the maxillary incisors?	Remove the incisors and reset new ones in wax and reassess Remove the incisors and reset new ones in wax and reassess

dentures; one such adverse effect is gagging or retching. Patients who experience gagging may be managed in a variety of ways. The fact that there are a variety of recommended ways indicates that there is no one way that can guarantee a successful outcome. Desensitisation programmes may be instituted which involve the patient being more in control of their problem. Patients may be encouraged to use a soft toothbrush to brush the area of the palate behind the upper incisors and to make a mark on the shank of the brush at the point where they are most comfortable, i.e. no retch reflex is induced. Over a period of days the insertion of the brush into the mouth can be progressively increased and the mark remade. This enables a 'progress report' to be made which

may increase patient confidence in having the palate covered.

Alternative strategies to try are:

- Hypnosis
- The use of 'training plates' (see Fig. CS 3.3). Should tolerance be favourable, then teeth may be added in stages, the eventual aim being that of a complete denture with full palatal coverage to effect maximum retention
- The use of fixatives to maximise retention and potentially decrease any rocking movements that may aggravate the gagging response
- Management by a professional psychological counsellor. In certain units, access to a trained professional may allow an appropriate

assessment and subsequent management of pyschological problems suffered by patients.

OTHER PROBLEM AREAS

Other problems pertaining to the review of patients with complete dentures may relate to the health of the oral tissues, such as:

- Burning mouth syndrome
- Denture stomatitis/angular cheilitis
- Allergy
- Temporomandibular joint disorders.

Burning mouth syndrome (BMS)

BMS has generated much interest, especially concerning its aetiology. There are many reported causes and the opinion of a specialist in oral medicine may be of value, especially to the patient, as the causes are seldom related to the dentures alone.

Denture stomatitis

As with BMS, denture stomatitis may have causes other than those directly under the control of the prosthodontist. It is prudent to provide the patient with dentures which are appropriate for them and ensure that they are being cleaned adequately. Prescription of an appropriate antifungal agent, e.g. a miconazole gel preparation for use in the impression or fitting surface of the dentures, may also be considered (NB: in the case of patients who are receiving anticoagulant agents such as warfarin, the patient's medical practitioner should be consulted as to the appropriate choice of anti-fungal agent) and a review appointment made. Where the above treatment does not result in the resolution of the problem, a referral to a specialist in oral medicine may be considered.

Allergy

There is little evidence in the literature as to the prevalence of true allergy to denture materials. It is apparently extremely rare and, where suspected, can be managed in conjunction with a dermatologist. Alternative denture materials may be considered, such as 'Luxene' (polycarbonate based) or nylon.

Temporomandibular dysfunction disorders (TMD)

TMDs and their relation to denture wearing have not been investigated sufficiently for any appropriate treatment protocol to be recommended. All that the prosthodontist may do is to prescribe dentures of appropriate design. Other treatments may be considered, such as jaw rest, a soft diet, TENS, physiotherapy or even medication, but the number of different treatment modalities does indicate that their success may not be guaranteed, and the patient should be thus informed.

MAINTENANCE

Maintenance of dentures is essential if continued oral health is to be monitored to allow any active intervention to be carried out if necessary. At the review appointment it is possible for the compliance of the patient to be assessed, and an inspection made of the mouth and masticatory apparatus. The optimum time for recall has not been established from evidence-based information, and in the opinion of the authors is best arranged according to the needs of the patient.

In addition, the review appointment allows the effect of denture wearing on any continuing alveolar resorption to be assessed, for example:

- Increasing instability of the appliance, causing difficulties with function, speech or comfort
- Relative overextension of the dentures, potentially resulting in tissue overgrowth
- Loss of satisfactory occlusal contacts.

The loss of fit may also be ascertained, and whereas in the past the authors considered the use of relining procedures, this would not now be considered an option. With any prosthesis, if there is the possibility of leaving it alone this should be the approach taken, as the patient may always revert to it should other treatment prove unsuccessful. In cases where correction of the fit surface is considered necessary, the use a replica technique is perceived to be more appropriate.

It has been advocated that dentures should be removed at night to permit the tissues of the oral cavity:

- To recover from the physical trauma of wearing the dentures
- To receive some stimulation from the tongue and the beneficial effect of contact with saliva
- To be relieved from contact with plaque and debris on the appliance.

There is undoubtedly an argument in favour of leaving the dentures out at night; however, most patients report that they do not do so for social reasons. This being the case, it must be emphasised that impeccable oral hygiene procedures must be exercised.

With respect to oral hygiene, a whole host of different advice and techniques seem to be recommended, but the regimen adopted by the authors is as follows:

- Use of a small-headed brush to clean all the surfaces of the denture, which is best demonstrated to the patient.
- The use of a non-abrasive agent such as household soap. The use of abrasive dentifices is not advisable as the surface polish of the denture may become roughened, encouraging the accumulation of plaque, debris and staining.
- Encourage the patient to hold the denture in a manner that reduces the possibility of breaking

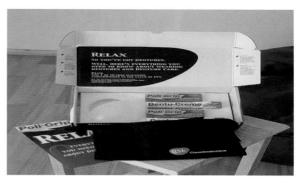

Fig. 6.7 It is useful to give patients kits such as this to encourage them in good denture maintenance.

it, and in addition to clean them over a bowl of water to lessen the blow if the denture is inadvertently dropped.

- Soak the dentures in a dilute solution of hypochlorite for 10 minutes and then rinse them in running water before inserting into the mouth (Fig. 6.7).
- Avoidance of placement of the dentures in hot water ($>70°C$), as this may cause them to whiten.

Occasionally the patient may need to be seen before or after the scheduled recall visit, for example if the denture fractures, there is discomfort of the mouth, or if there is a marked deterioration in function.

REFERENCE

McCord JF, Grant AA, Quayle AA. Treatment options for the edentulous mandible. Eur J Prosthodont Rest Dent 1992; I: 19–23

7 Technological aspects of complete denture-making

This chapter is not intended to present a detailed description of the dental technology relevant to complete denture construction. Rather, it is intended to present a précis of each technical stage to enable interested readers to be aware of what to look for so that acceptable prosthodontic outcomes might be achieved. For this reason, the chapter will address the production of casts and special trays, the production of rims and trial dentures and, finally, processing and preparing dentures for delivery.

PRODUCING CASTS AND SPECIAL TRAYS

In order for complete dentures to be constructed the dental technician needs to have casts of the edentulous areas on which to make the prostheses. The dentures themselves are constructed with the fitting surface made on a definitive cast, which represents the denture-bearing tissues recorded by the clinician. As was indicated in Chapter 3, in order to record the supporting tissues appropriately it is preferable to have two separate appointments for impression-making: one for the primary impression and the other for definitive impressions.

Impressions are typically poured in fluid gypsum-based products which, on setting, produce casts of the mouth on which subsequent technical procedures may be carried out. It should be evident that, as in all clinical procedures, there is a need to handle impressions appropriately and ensure that they have been decontaminated prior to despatch to the laboratory. The first task the technician has to perform is to prepare primary casts.

Primary casts are principally used to provide bases on which customised or 'special' impression trays are constructed. In addition, they are also useful in planning treatment, for example when outlining the potential supporting areas of the denture-bearing tissues.

Adequate primary casts may be poured in a 50:50 mixture of dental stone/plaster of Paris vacuum-mixed with the manufacturer's recommended volume of water. The impressions are best cast using vibration to eliminate air bubbles, which might otherwise adversely affect the surface detail or strength of the casts. The cast should preferably record the width of the sulci and be surrounded by a sufficient 'land' width, as this facilitates the outlining and construction of the special tray. It is recommended that the base should be 10 mm thicker than the deepest part of the impression. Thinner bases may be insufficiently robust to survive subsequent handling and laboratory procedures; ones that are significantly thicker (in master casts) may be difficult to

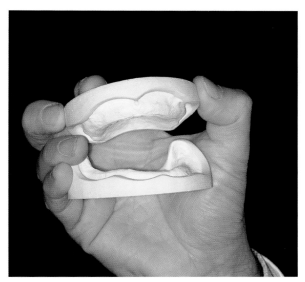

Fig. 7.1 Well-prepared primary casts.

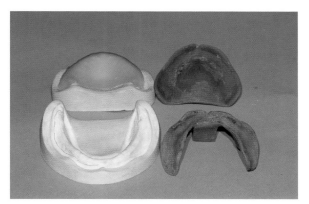

Fig. 7.2 This maxillary tray has had 2 mm spacing and the mandibular tray is close fitting.

accommodate in an articulator or denture flasks used in processing (Fig. 7.1).

Special trays

These should be made to follow the clinical prescription, which should stipulate the following:

- Material to be used in the construction of the tray
- The amount of spacing to be used on the primary cast and therefore incorporated into the special tray (Fig. 7.2)
- Handles designed to avoid distorting the lips, and/or positioned to act as finger rests (Fig. 7.3)
- The tray should cover the entire denture-bearing area but should ideally finish just short of the sulcus to provide space for border moulding (Fig. 7.4).

Summaries of guidelines for casts and customised trays are given in Tables 7.1 and 7.2.

RIMS AND TRIAL DENTURES

The requirements of rims and their form were discussed in Chapter 4. This section will therefore specify the placement of teeth on the trial

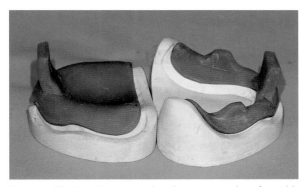

Fig. 7.3 The handles are so placed so as not to interfere with lip positioning during recording of the definitive impressions.

Table 7.1 Summary of technical guidelines for casts

Features	Primary casts	Working casts
Materials	Plaster/stone (50:50)	Dental stone
Base thickness	1 cm greater than deepest part of impression	1 cm thicker than deepest part of impression
Land area	Always recorded	Always recorded
Sulci	Full width and depth preserved by marking 'peripheral roll' on preliminary impression	Full width and depth preserved by 'boxing in' peripheral roll on definitive impression

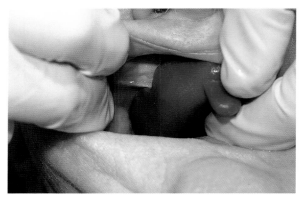

Fig. 7.4 The periphery of the tray should not be overextended.

Table 7.2 Summary of technical guidelines for special trays

Features	Special tray
Material	Rigid, e.g. visible light-cured resin
Spacer	Wax thickness depends on impression material/technique
Handles	'Stub' sited to take account of support/technique
Extent	Cover entire denture-bearing area, 2 mm short of sulcus to facilitate border moulding

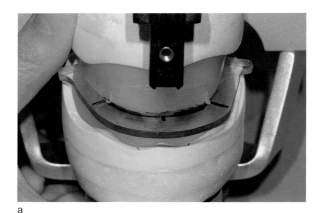

a

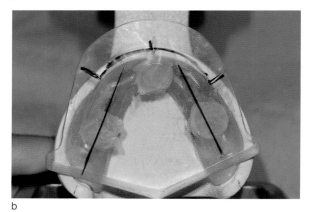

b

Fig. 7.5 (a) The form of the labial arc has been scribed on to the translucent plate. (b) The relative position of the mandibular ridge has been indicated on the translucent plate.

dentures, and specifically regular set-ups; for details of other characterised tooth placements, readers are referred to other texts (Winkler 1988, Zarb et al. 1990). In keeping with the context of the clinical stages, the placement of teeth will be considered in two sections, namely placement of anterior teeth and placement of posterior teeth. To ensure that placement of the maxillary teeth conforms to the outline of the maxillary rim or aesthetic control base, a transparent mounting plate may be used and this may also be used later to assist in the placement of maxillary posterior teeth (Fig.7.5a and b).

Placement of anterior teeth

Maxillary central incisors should be placed such that their labial faces conform to the outline of the

rim (Fig. 7.6). The long axes of these teeth should be such that they lie 5° to the vertical (pregrinding of the palatal cingulum/cervical area is therefore probably necessary); when viewed from the side, the tips are therefore more labially placed than the necks.

Maxillary lateral incisors, when viewed face-on, should have an inclination of their long axes 7° from the vertical. Ideally, their incisal edges should be 1–1.5 mm above the level of the central incisors.

Maxillary canines are the keystones of the arch, as they link the anterior teeth with the posterior teeth. When viewed from the side, the canine ridge of each tooth, indicating the long axis, is vertical; when viewed from face-on, the neck should be out slightly to commence the buccal corridors (Figs 7.7, 7.8). When the set-up is viewed from

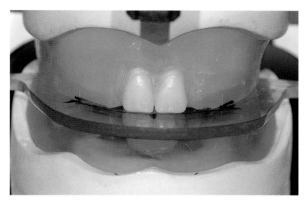

Fig. 7.6 Appropriate placement of the maxillary central incisors.

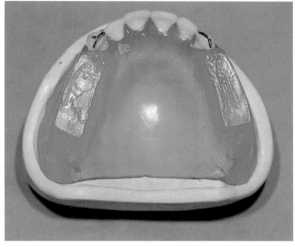

Fig. 7.9 Occlusal view of maxillary anterior teeth.

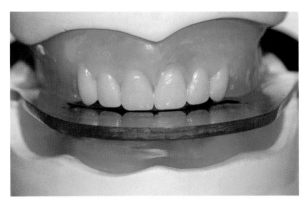

Fig. 7.7 Face-on view of maxillary incisor and canine teeth.

the occlusal view (Fig. 7.9), the smaller anterior third of each canine imparts an anterior component to the set-up, whereas the larger posterior component points towards the posterior set-up. This view is useful as it may point out asymmetries relative to the midline (Fig. 7.10).

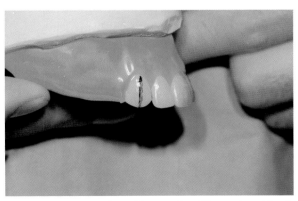

Fig. 7.8 Side view of maxillary canine. The canine ridge is vertical.

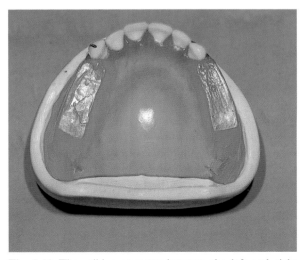

Fig. 7.10 The mild asymmetry between the left and right sides is illustrated here.

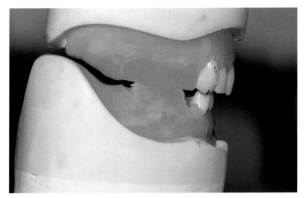

Fig. 7.11 Placement of mandibular incisor and canine teeth must conform to the aesthetic and functional needs of the patient.

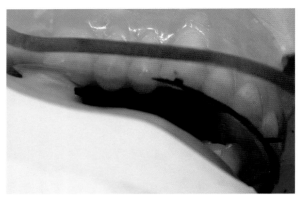

Fig. 7.12 The palatal cusps of the maxillary premolar teeth are contacting the plate where it marks the relative position of the mandibular ridge.

Mandibular anterior teeth

Although the relative positions of these teeth may be altered after placement of the posterior teeth, they should nevertheless obey certain prosthodontic norms. For example, they should be set up with their necks over the residual ridges and their tips slightly labial to the ridge. Their absolute placement, however, depends on the occlusal and muscular preferences of each patient (Fig. 7.11).

Placement of posterior teeth

The maxillary premolars and molars must, like the mandibular anterior teeth, conform to the aesthetic and functional needs of the patient. With the Perspex mounting rim in place, the maxillary premolars should be set with their long axes parallel to the canines and with their necks out, again to create the potential for the inclusion of buccal corridors. The palatal cusps should contact the mounting plate where it marks the relative position of the mandibular ridge (Fig. 7.12). The same is true for the mandibular molars, although some consideration should be given to the compensating curves by raising all but the mesiopalatal cusps of the maxillary molars off the plate (Fig. 7.13).

The mandibular teeth are set up usually with the first molars in the first place. As we aspire to balanced articulation, the mandibular first molar teeth should interdigitate closely with the opposing teeth. In RCP, the maxillary anterior buccal cusp should lie between the mandibular buccal cusps. In protrusion, the anterior and posterior buccal cusps of each mandibular first molar tooth should contact the buccal cusp of the maxillary second premolar and the mesiobuccal cusp of the maxillary first molar, respectively (Fig. 7.14). In (left) working occlusion the teeth should conform to the cuspal position indicated in Figure 7.15, whereas balancing contacts should conform to the relationship illustrated in Figure 7.16. The reader at this stage requires an understanding of mandibular movements and an awareness of the influence that condylar movement will have on the arrangement of the teeth in complete dentures, especially with regard to balanced articulation.

After the posterior teeth are set up to conform to the occlusal needs of the patient, the mandibular incisors may need to be altered to conform to the functional requirements of the dentures.

The final artistic touch is related to the waxwork, and this may make or break the appearance of a denture. In general, the waxwork around a tooth may be considered the gingival matrix, and it must in general satisfy three constraints:

- Be convex anteroposteriorly and mesiodistally
- Have appropriate form of the gingival curves and at appropriate cervical heights

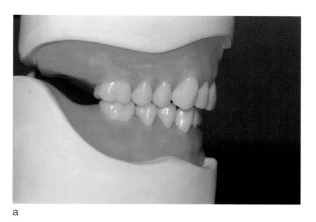

a

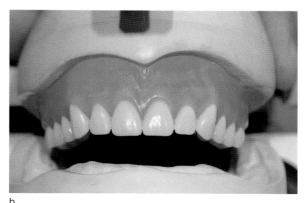

b

Fig. 7.13 The anteroposterior and buccopalatal compensating curves have been incorporated in the maxillary molar.

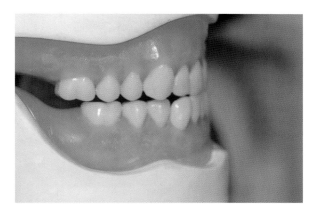

Fig. 7.14 Side view of try-in in protrusion.

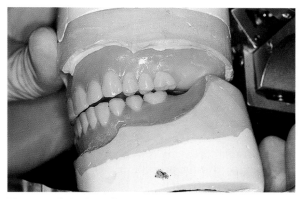

Fig. 7.15 Side view of try-in in right working.

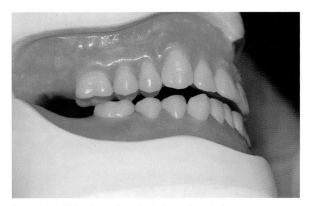

Fig. 7.16 Side view of try-in balanced articulation.

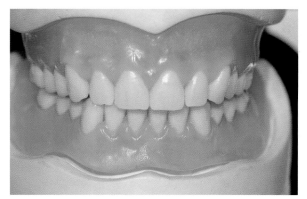

Fig. 7.17 Good gingival architecture.

- Have appropriately formed and well demarcated interdental papilla; the effects of sloppy technological work can be distressing.

PROCESSING AND PREPARING DENTURES FOR DELIVERY

Processing

On completion the wax trial dentures should be carefully sealed to both the upper and the lower casts at their peripheries while they are still mounted on the articulator. The casts and trial dentures are then separated from the mounting plaster (they are 'joined' either by indexing or magnets, so that they may be rearticulated after processing). The trial dentures are then ready for flasking – so called as they are placed in flasks to have the wax replaced precisely with the permanent denture base. The flasks have two halves, one shallower than the other (see below). The cast and trial denture for each arch are placed in the shallower portion of the flask (Fig. 7.18), leaving sufficient area for the investment plaster to hold them in position. The investment plaster is brought up to the periphery of the trial denture and with the lower, care should be made to ensure that the retromolar areas are fully supported to prevent any damage during processing, as in some cases these areas may be delicate (Fig. 7.19).

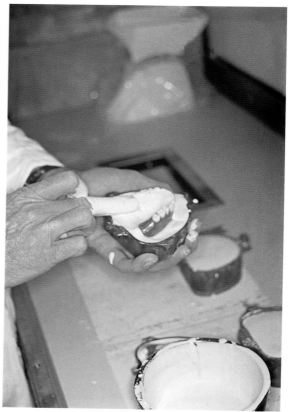

Fig. 7.19 Here the gypsum mix is applied over the denture prior to placing the upper or topping half of the flask.

After investing, the plaster should be left to set and dry out completely. Once set, the investment plaster should be coated with a suitable separating medium, e.g. sodium silicate. Once the separator has dried and any excess moisture has been removed, the 'topping' procedure can be carried out. A vacuum mix of 50% plaster/kaffir D is prepared and a thin preinvestment coat is applied to the teeth and gingival areas of the wax-up. At this stage great care should be exercised to avoid any air being trapped around these areas, otherwise defects might be incorporated in the processed dentures. The reason the deeper portion is used to house the teeth is to give greater resistance to packing pressure and so prevent movement of the denture teeth.

After preinvesting, the opposing flask should be carefully assembled and the remaining topping

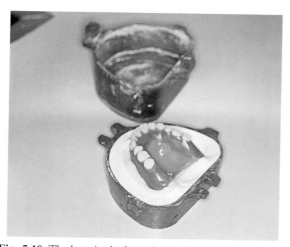

Fig. 7.18 The base in the lower half of the flask.

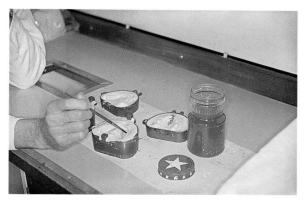

Fig. 7.20 The flask opened up and removal of wax. A separating medium is being applied on the investing gypsum.

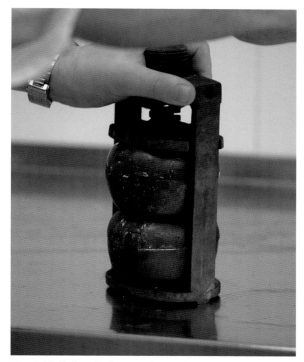

Fig. 7.21 Before final processing a trial packing is performed and then the flasks are subjected to pressure in a spring-loaded clamp.

mix used to fill the flasks, again avoiding any air trapping. Once the topping plaster has set, the flasks should be placed in boiling water for approximately 8–10 minutes to allow the flasks to be adequately heat-soaked. The flasks may then be separated and the (softened) wax removed with running boiling water (Fig. 7.20). It is essential that this stage be carried out thoroughly to ensure that no residual wax is left on either the fitting or the non-fitting surfaces, as this could result in a poor chemical bond between the acrylic and the denture teeth. After boiling out, the flasks should be left to cool and then the flask containing the teeth should be coated with an isolating liquid to prevent the topping plaster adhering to the acrylic. Once the isolating liquid has dried, the denture base may be prepared. Conventionally, acrylic resin (PMMA) is used in the form of monomer and polymer, although a cross-linking agent such as ethylene glycol dimethacrylate may be incorporated. The acrylic should be mixed according to the manufacturer's instructions.

When the mix is at the 'dough' stage it is ready to pack into the mould. Sufficient acrylic should be placed in the half of the flask containing the teeth and a polythene separating sheet placed on top. The two flasks are then assembled, placed in a press and gently squeezed to allow any excess acrylic to extrude (Fig. 7.21). Once the flasks are fully closed without any excess visible, they should be removed from the press and carefully opened. The moulds may then be examined to ensure that

there are no underpacked areas. If there are any deficiencies, additional material should be added and the packing procedure redone. The separating sheet should be left in place while the flask containing the model is coated with the same isolating liquid to prevent the acrylic drying out. Before final closure, the separating sheet should be removed and any visible excess of acrylic trimmed with a sharp instrument. The flasks should then be carefully assembled and returned to the press for final closure (usually 100 bar pressure). Following this, the assembly is processed according to the manufacturer's instructions.

Alternative materials may used for the denture base, such as polycarbonate where an allergy or suspected allergy to acrylic is present. The process for these materials does not differ from that described above.

A technological development considered to result in superior processing of the dentures is that

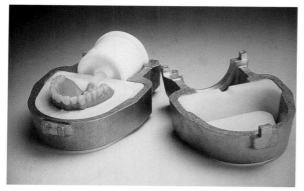

Fig. 7.22 As in Figure 7.18, the maxillary denture is mounted in the lower half of the cast.

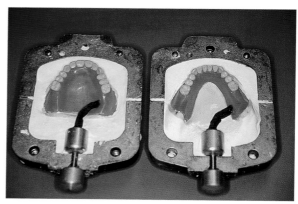

Fig. 7.24 Flasks opened prior to removal of wax. Note the sprues for the PMMA to be injected.

of injection-moulding. The principle of investing is the same as above, but with the addition of wax sprues attached to the posterior borders of both upper and lower wax trial dentures. The flasks used accommodate these sprues when assembled (Fig. 7.22). Topping-up of the flask is similar to conventional processing (Fig. 7.23). The boiling-out process (Fig. 7.24) and the application of isolating liquid are similar to the conventional method, with the difference being the mode of introduction of the acrylic resin. This is performed by assembling the flasks and placing them in a press driven by compressed air (Fig. 7.24). A cartridge containing premixed acrylic is attached

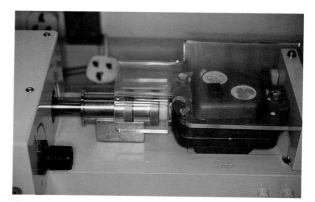

Fig. 7.25 Flask in the injection-moulding machine.

to the flask and aligned with the sprues, and then the mixture is injection into the mould by compressed air (Fig. 7.25). Once the injection is completed, the processed denture is taken out and the sprues removed (Fig. 7.26). Processing then progresses as outlined above and for the duration recommended by the manufacturer.

Finishing or polishing the dentures

When the processing cycle has been completed the flasks should be removed from the processing unit, as processing temperatures can reach up to (but should not exceed) 100°C. The flasks should

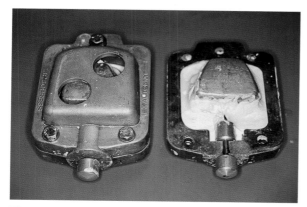

Fig. 7.23 Topping-up is taking place.

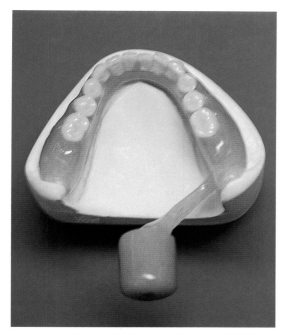

Fig. 7.26 Processed denture prior to removal of sprue and polishing.

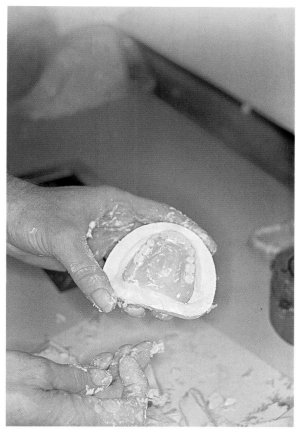

Fig. 7.27 After curing the flasks are opened up and the dentures plus their bases are carefully removed.

be allowed to cool naturally and not plunged into cold water, as this could result in warping of the denture bases, as could removal of the dentures when the moulds are still hot. Once cool, the plaster moulds should be removed from the flasks carefully (Fig. 7.27) and, where possible, intact (en bloc). Use of careful saw-cuts into the plaster mould should result in its easy removal from the processed denture. Any remaining plaster should be removed from the denture, which may then be returned to the mounting plaster and mounted on the articulator by the indices or magnetic means of location (Fig. 7.28).

This procedure allows the occlusion to be checked and any required adjustment to the teeth performed with some confidence. The dentures may then be removed from the casts. Finishing is then progressed by removing any excess acrylic around the peripheral areas of the dentures, using acrylic trimming burs, taking care not to remove any vital areas such as the peripheral roll and postdam. The non-fitting surfaces of the dentures

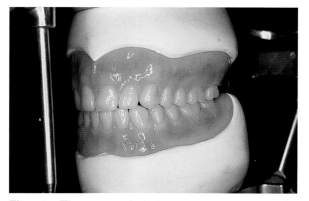

Fig. 7.28 The processed dentures are now ready to be remounted to review the occlusion.

can be smoothed with silicone-mounted polishers. The fitting surfaces should be inspected for any obvious imperfections but should not be polished. On completion of these modifications, the dentures are then ready for polishing. The first stage is to use a coarse mop and pumice on all non-fitting surfaces to remove any obvious bur marks or abrasions. Then a finer mop or bristle brush is used with a thinner consistency of pumice and water, and then finally a very fine brush is used. Great care must be taken during the polishing process to ensure that no damage occurs to any tooth surfaces: critical areas to protect are the labial surfaces of the anterior teeth and the buccal, occlusal, palatal and lingual surfaces of the posterior teeth.

The dentures are then washed to remove any remaining pumice, dried, and checked for any abrasive or brush marks. After this, the dentures are ready to receive the final high-gloss finish (Fig. 7.29). This is achieved typically by the use of a soft white mop and an acrylic gloss compound, e.g. tripoli. Care should be taken to apply this evenly to avoid burning the acrylic. Once completed, the dentures should be washed and once again carefully checked for any defects. They are then sealed in a moist polythene bag prior to delivery to the clinician, to prevent drying out.

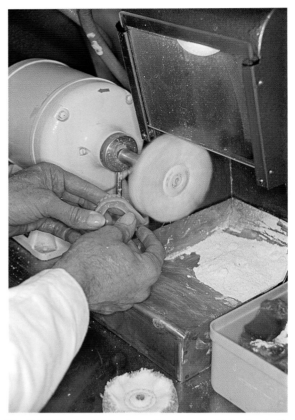

Fig. 7.29 Final polishing is used to impart a high gloss to the surface.

REFERENCES

Winkler S. Complete denture prosthodontics, 2nd edn. St Louis: Mosby, 1988

Zarb GA, Bolender CL, Hickey JC, Carlsson GE. Boucher's prosthodontic treatment for edentulous patients, 10th edn. St Louis: Mosby, 1990

Case Study 1: Copy or template technique

Mrs K. H. – Age 73 years

Occupation	Housewife
Past medical history	Angina brought on after walking several hundred yards or up a few flights of stairs. Hypertension, 'slight' stroke 1987.
Medication	Aspirin, amlodipine, GTN spray
Social history	Lives at home with her husband
Dental history	Extraction of natural teeth approximately 40 years ago followed by provision of complete immediate dentures. Four sets of dentures in this time, including the most recent ones. Sought replacement dentures because previous ones were loose and worn.
Complaint	'doesn't talk right with new dentures', and 'mouth feels too full when wearing new dentures'.
Clinical assessment	Spectacle wearer with apparent left-sided partial palsy resulting from previous stroke. Hearing aid worn in the left ear. 'Whistling' was clearly evident on speaking and patient obviously needed to make a concerted effort to obtain lip seal when enunciating plosive sounds. Maxillary and mandibular edentulous ridges were well formed and rounded. Muscle tone on the left side was lower than on the right side. Features noted in the most recent C/C compared with previously worn C/C: 1. C/– occlusal plane set too low (Fig. CS 1.1) 2. Incisal relationship edge to edge (Fig. CS 1.2) 3. Excessive occlusal vertical dimension negative freeway space –3 mm.

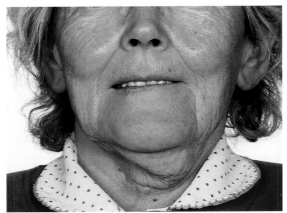

Fig. CS 1.1 Facial view of previous denture preferred by patient.

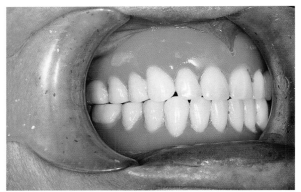

Fig. CS 1.2 Occlusal relationship of the denture seen in Figure CS 1.1.

Comments

1. The amount of reduction in occlusal vertical dimension is on the limit of reasonable accuracy without recourse to removing teeth and replacing them with registration rims. Leaving the tooth position unaltered would do nothing to improve speech, and similarly retention would not be improved.

2. Making new dentures is a possibility but there is a risk that, given the patient's history of a stroke and palsy, she might experience difficulty in adapting to and tolerating new dentures.

3. Relining/rebasing the previous dentures would improve the fit and retention but would do nothing to address the patient's complaints about wear. There is also a significant risk that should the relining procedure be unsuccessful the patient would be worse off, as she might be unable to wear prostheses that she had been comfortable with until that time.

4. Using the previous dentures as a template for the incorporation of appropriate modifications is an attractive option. It allows the well-tolerated tooth position and polished surface contours to be reproduced while allowing for improvements in fit and renewal of the worn artificial teeth. This would address the complaints regarding changes in speech and tolerance the patient had experienced with her most recent dentures, together with those of looseness and wear regarding the previous ones.

Treatment options

1. Remove and reset teeth on most recent dentures following facebow recording and occlusal registration of RCP
2. Conventional replacement complete dentures with appropriate freeway space
3. Template ('copy') dentures aiming to maintain arch form, polished surface contour and tooth position
4. Reline/rebase procedure for old dentures.

Treatment agreed

Provision of template dentures aimed at:

1. Preserving polished surface contours, particularly the palatal aspect of the upper denture and generally of the lower denture (speech and adaptation) plus tooth position (speech)

2. Improvement in peripheral, postdam seal and fit via modification of the denture peripheries and wash impressions
3. Minimal increase in occlusal vertical dimension to compensate for wear of occlusal surfaces and alveolar resorption.

The new dentures were provided, copying those with which the patient could cope, and the patient reported that she was able to speak and eat as before but with enhanced retention of her new dentures (Figs CS1.3, 1.4). The tooth positioning was confirmed with an Alma gauge (Fig. CS1.5).

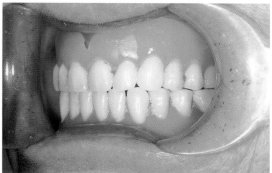

Fig. CS 1.3 Completed template denture illustrating similar occlusal relationship.

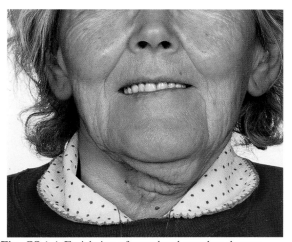

Fig. CS 1.4 Facial view of completed template denture.

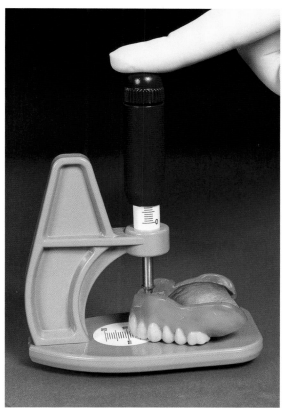

Fig. CS 1.5 The tooth positioning was verified with an Alma gauge.

Case Study 2: Very worn old C/C

Mr J. R. – Age 55 years

Occupation	Engineer
Past medical history	NAD
Social history	NAD
Dental history	Had been edentulous for 12 years and had worn two pairs of dentures, one pair immediate dentures and a replacement pair which was 11 years old.
Complaint	Main problems were wear of the occlusal and polished surfaces of both dentures and of 'looking older than my years' (Figs CS2.1 and CS2.2).
Clinical assessment	Mild angular cheilitis, Atwood IV order of ridges in all sextants, excessive freeway space, mandibular ridge tender on digital palpation of that ridge.

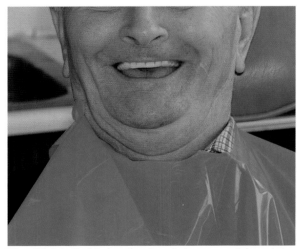

Fig. CS 2.1 Facial view showing obvious wear of the existing maxillary denture. The mandibular denture was not visible.

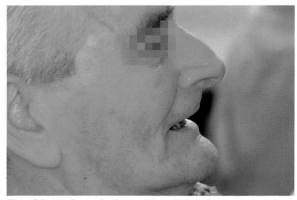

Fig. CS 2.2 Lateral view with existing dentures in place. Note the lack of maxillary lip support.

Treatment options

1. Do nothing
2. Reline complete upper/complete lower dentures (C/C)
3. Replace C/C conventionally
4. Replica or template dentures
5. Replace C/C with transitional dentures in the first instance and thereafter make replacement dentures
6. Implant – retained –/C plus C/– (conventional or implant-retained).

Discussion

1. Neither what the patient wants nor is it desirable.
2. May address the problem of the lack of fit of the impression surfaces but addresses neither the problems of the occlusal surfaces nor the problem of insufficient OVD.
3. Possible, but two factors of relevance here, namely the narrowness of the existing occlusal table might cause problems of adjusting to the conventional cuspal architecture, and secondly the need to avoid embarrassment to the patient, as providing what might be perceived to be prosthodontically acceptable dentures might cause comments on what may appear to be an obvious new denture.
4. Replica or template dentures are an option, but no current replica technique can adequately deal with support problems where selective impression techniques are required.
5. This was the option chosen by the patient, as it offered a good intermediate phase that in no way altered his current denture, yet offered the potential to improve both his appearance and his eating ability.
6. The patient was made aware of this option but did not perceive a need for it at this time, denture wearing not being a major problem to him.

Treatment offered

Replace C/C with transitional dentures in the first instance and thereafter make replacement dentures.

Stages

1. Use of a replica technique to 'copy' the polished surfaces of present C/C (see Case Study 1), with the modifications being that a selective impression technique was used for the mandibular denture using greenstick tracing compound, relieving the impression over the ridge and refining the impression using light-bodied poly(vinyl)siloxane (McCord & Grant 2000) and that the wax was added to the labial surfaces to restore the tooth support to the lips (Figs CS 2.3, 2.4).
2. Use of occlusal pivots to increase OVD and yet offer a small, flat occlusal table to permit the patient to 'find' RCP (Fig. 2.5).
3. When the patient had adapted to the transitional dentures, conventional replacement dentures were made, again using the selected pressure technique described above (Figs. CS 2.6, 2.7a, 2.7b).

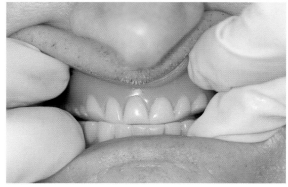

Fig. CS 2.3 The wear of the existing dentures is apparent here.

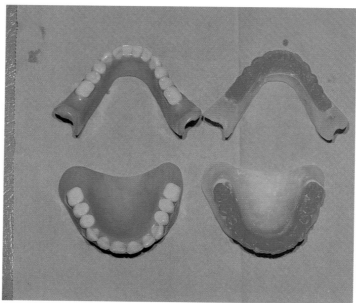

Fig. CS 2.4 Templates or replicas of the existing dentures are shown alongside the 'old dentures'. The occlusal surfaces have been replicated in wax.

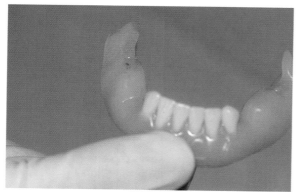

Fig. CS 2.5 Replicated transitional mandibular denture which has a tissue conditioner lining.

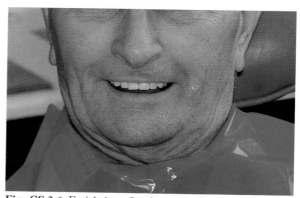

Fig. CS 2.6 Facial view of replacement dentures at insertion.

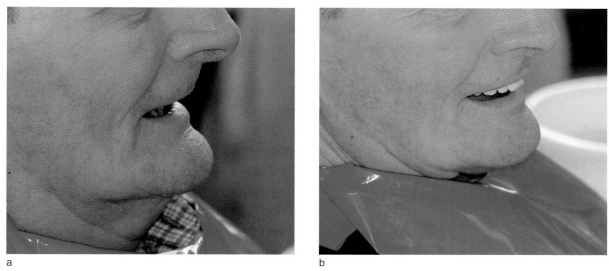

a   b

Fig. CS 2.7 (a) Side view of 'old' dentures in place. (b) Side view with replacement dentures in place one week post insertion.

Case Study 3: Gagging/denture intolerance

Mr S. B. – Age 55 years

Occupation	Lorry driver
Past medical history	Irritable bowel syndrome; takes sleeping tablets Lorazepam 2 mg
Social history	Admits to smoking 12 cigarettes per day
Dental history	Was prescribed a maxillary partial denture 5 years previously and had been able to wear it for 'up to a couple of hours at a time'. His remaining teeth were extracted 6 months ago.
Complaint	Very concerned that he cannot tolerate the maxillary denture for 'any more than a minute', although the –/C is tolerated.
Clinical assessment	Mucosa appears healthy, Atwood III order of ridges in all sextants. Patient did not retch when (gloved) forefinger was used to palpate ridge or when postdam area was lightly palpated.

Treatment options

1. Do nothing
2. Replace C/C conventionally and hope for the best
3. Use a desensitisation technique, supply a training plate and make replacement dentures
4. Implant-retained prosthesis.

Discussion

1. Not desired by patient or his family.
2. May work, although it is most unlikely that the patient will be able to undertake the impression techniques, the stages leading to replacement dentures, and thereafter to be able to wear the dentures.
3. This was the option chosen by the patient as it offered a means of desensitising the palate allowing (hopefully – there is never a guarantee of success here) good adjustment to a training plate prior to the provision of a replacement denture similar in form to the end-stage of the training plate.
4. The patient was not interested in having surgery carried out. He also had no intention in stopping smoking.

Treatment offered

Use a desensitisation technique, supply a training plate and make replacement dentures.

Stages

1. Show patient how to massage palate only to first joint of the forefinger (may also add toothpaste to finger) of the hand the patient prefers to use, moving it from side to side gently. Patient informed not to advance any more than the first joint for a

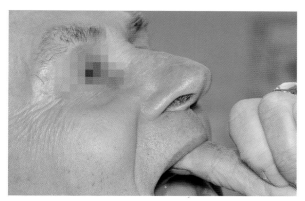

Fig. CS 3.1 The palate is palpated up to the first joint of the finger (here the patient is using his left thumb).

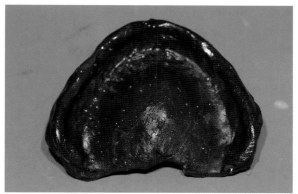

Fig. CS 3.2 The definitive impression has been recorded in greenstick tracing compound, which sets within 30 seconds of insertion.

week (Fig. CS 3.1). After review at 1 week, the clinician should assess whether the patient can advance to halfway between the first and second joints. The aim is to progress to the second joint of the forefinger, and it must be emphasised to the patient that this is not a rapid process and that speed is not a necessity.

2. After 4–6 weeks the patient is asked to demonstrate progress; if sufficient coverage of the palate may be 'massaged' by the patient, then the clinician may proceed to prepare the training plate; if not, further time may be required or, indeed, other techniques may be required, such as temporal tamponade, relaxation therapy or hypnosis.

Impression compound is recommended for the recording of the primary impression, as this may be controlled for extension, does not flow copiously, and may be removed from the mouth after 30 seconds. A special tray may then be made and the definitive impression recorded in greenstick tracing compound, for similar reasons to those for impression compound, although the latter is much less viscous than the former (Fig. CS3.2) On the resultant master cast, a wax trial training plate or training denture may be created with the six maxillary teeth in place and with reduced palatal coverage (Fig. CS3.3). When the tooth positions are agreed, the

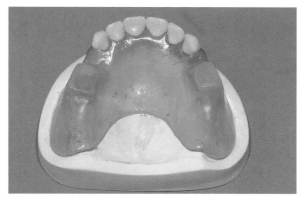

Fig. CS 3.3 Wax registration rim showing extension of denture base.

registration is recorded, via the patient's present –/C. The training plate is processed with only six anterior teeth, small occlusal platforms bilaterally and a minimally extended palate (Fig. CS3.4). This plate must exhibit balanced occlusion in RCP but, as a flat occlusal platform is provided in the maxillary second premolar area, balanced articulation cannot be achieved; consequently, the patient must be advised that it is most likely that a denture fixative will be required, and this aspect of care will be addressed in another Case Study.

3. The patient is assessed to determine progress with the training plate; if he still complains of retching, the plate may have

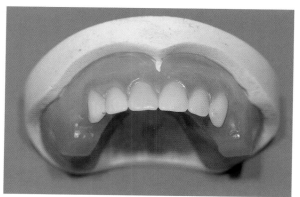

Fig. CS 3.4 Frontal view of trial denture.

to be reduced in extension, although this will further aggravate the inherent problems of retention and (in)stability: if further problems persist, referral to a specialist in prosthodontics may be the best option. If the patient is coping well, then the treatment options are either to accept the status quo, to make a definite denture via a replica technique, or to attempt, gradually, to extend the training plate via the use of as chairside relining material.

4. When a satisfactory outcome has been achieved, the training plate and the existing –/C are replicated using the technique described in Case Study 1.

Case Study 4: Denture stomatitis

Mrs S. W. – Age 85 years

Occupation	Retired schoolteacher
Past medical history	Nil relevant
Social history	Non-smoker
Dental history	Lost the majority of her teeth in adolescence as a result of periodontal disease. Has worn maxillary and mandibular complete dentures successfully for 50 years. Four sets of dentures had been fabricated in those 50 years and the most recent set were 10 years old.
Complaint	Patient had noticed reddening of the palate and at the commissures of the mouth which were 'becoming sore'. The dentures were considered satisfactory by the patient.
Clinical assessment	The mucosa of the palate under the denture appeared reddened (Fig. CS 4.1). Examination of the dentures revealed that hygiene was very poor, with generalised plaque and food deposits. The retention of the maxillary denture was normatively considered to be less than ideal, but the patient felt that they were satisfactory. The angles of the mouth were reddened and cracked (Fig. CS 4.2). A diagnosis of denture stomatitis and angular cheilitis was made. It was considered that the aetiology was multifactorial, with the possible causes being:

1. Poor denture hygiene
2. Wearing of dentures all day and night
3. Poorly fitting dentures
4. Underlying systemic upset – haematological, diabetes, immunological.

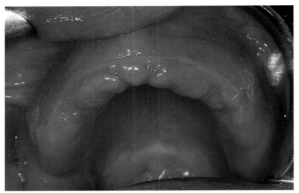

Fig. CS 4.1 The mucosa over the denture-bearing area is clearly inflamed.

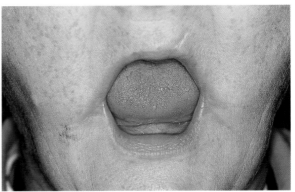

Fig. CS 4.2 There is marked angular cheilitis evident here.

Treatment options

1. Do nothing
2. Advise the patient to leave out the dentures all the time
3. Offer denture hygiene
4. Advise the use of miconazole gel applied to the fitting surface of the denture and review
5. Replace C/C
6. Consider a referral to an oral physician.

Discussion

Doing nothing was not considered appropriate as the patient had a complaint of soreness. In view of the very poor oral hygiene it was felt appropriate to offer oral hygiene advice and encourage the patient to leave the dentures out at night. The patient was later reviewed and the clinical situation had completely resolved. This case highlights the importance of treating the obvious first. There was no need to resort to medication, which was advantageous. In view of the fact that the dentures were being worn satisfactorily, it would have been inappropriate to consider remake or replica dentures at that stage, as any changes made in new dentures, however small, may still require some neuromuscular adaptation, and in an 85-year-old this could be somewhat problematic. Should the situation not have resolved, then consideration could have been given to pursuing the use of miconazole gel on the fitting surface of the denture: should this have not led to resolution, then a referral to an oral physician could have been made.

Case Study 5: Selective pressure impression technique

Mr H. A. – Age 68 years	
Occupation	Retired engineer
Past medical history	Asthma, bronchitis
Medication	Duovent and Flixotide inhalers
Social history	Lives at home with his wife
Dental history	Maxillary natural teeth and posterior mandibular teeth extracted approximately 35 years ago as a result of caries. During this time he has had four complete maxillary dentures. Initially he also had a mandibular partial denture, but this was never worn ('I just never could get on with it'); subsequently never wanted to have another partial denture.
Complaint	'Loose upper' denture, especially when eating
Clinical assessment	Maxillary denture-bearing area exhibited displaceable tissue in the anterior maxilla (Fig. CS 5.1). Oral hygiene and periodontal support for the remaining mandibular teeth was good, with only minimal gingival recession and no increased periodontal probing depths. The complete maxillary denture demonstrated poor retention, principally owing to a lack of peripheral and postdam seal. In addition, this denture was unstable and there was a marked premature contact in RCP (Fig. CS 5.2) with a subsequent slide into ICP (Fig. CS 5.3).

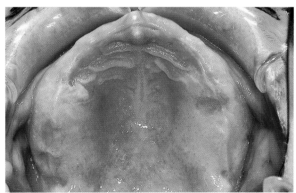

Fig. CS 5.1 Mirror view of patient's maxillary ridge. Note the indication of displaceable tissue anteriorly.

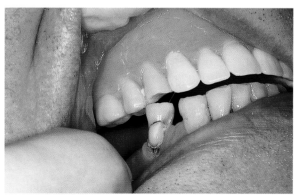

Fig. CS 5.2 There is an obvious occlusal prematurity on the patient's right in RCP.

	Encroachment of the cheeks and tongue virtually eliminated any potential mandibular denture space.
Charting	The remaining natural dentition comprised all six mandibular anterior teeth plus the two first mandibular premolars.

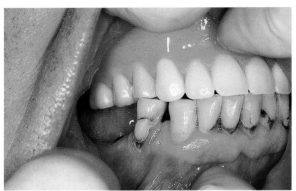

Fig. CS 5.3 Occlusal arrangement in ICP.

Treatment options

1. No active treatment
2. Reline existing maxillary denture
3. Provision of new maxillary denture and mandibular partial denture
4. Provision of new maxillary denture and bilateral distal cantilever bridges
5. Provision of implant-stabilised and retained maxillary prosthesis (fixed or removable).

Comments

1. Not a realistic option in this instance, given the patient's desire to be able to eat comfortably in the company of others.
2. Relining the existing C/– would improve retention, and if done appropriately also stability. This would not solve the problem posed by the occlusal instability resulting from the premature occlusal contact.
3. Replacing the C/– gives the potential to improve retention and stability and also ensure that occlusal imbalance is minimised. Providing a mandibular partial denture would be problematic given the

patient's previous intolerance to an RPD, together with his reluctance to wear one.
4. Replacing the C/– gives the potential advantages outlined in (3) above. Providing distal cantilever bridges gives the possibility of improved occlusal stability, together with current evidence that this form of restoration has good success in the medium term.
5. An implant-retained and stabilised upper prosthesis has the undoubted potential to provide a functionally superior result to the other options. However, in this case the patient declined any treatment that would involve elective surgery.

Treatment agreed

1. Provision of minimal preparation distal cantilever bridges carrying second premolar pontics from retainers on the first premolar abutments. Bridge retainers were designed to cover lingual cusps to provide improved retention and resistance form (Fig. CS 5.4).
2. New C/– via selective pressure impression to take account of displaceable tissue in the anterior maxilla while also ensuring an appropriate peripheral and postdam seal, to be achieved through careful border moulding (Fig. CS 5.5). A facebow record would be obtained to allow approximation of the arc of closure on the articulator with the hinge axis in the patient. Occlusion would be carefully recorded to ensure coincidence of RCP and ICP (Fig. CS 5.6 a and b). Cast gold metal occlusal surfaces were to be incorporated into maxillary first and second premolars (Fig. CS 5.7) in an attempt to maintain occlusal stability by reducing wear.

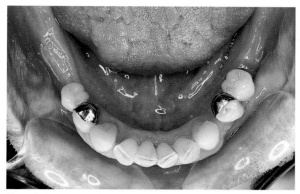

Fig. CS 5.4 Occlusal view of restored mandibular arch.

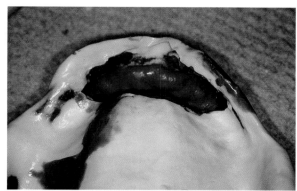

Fig. CS 5.5 View of completed impression using medium- and light-bodied PVS impression material for the selective-pressure impression technique.

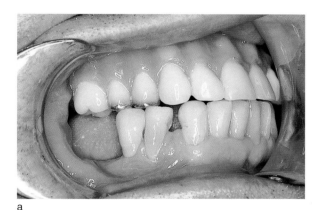

a

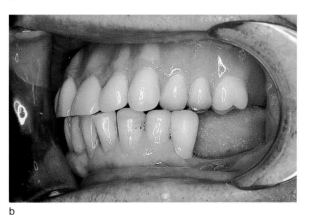

b

Fig. CS 5.6 (a) View of RCP, which is coincident with ICP in replacement denture. (b) The gold occlusal surfaces impart good occlusal stability and a not unpleasing appearance.

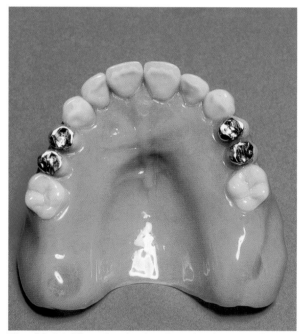

Fig. CS 5.7 View of occlusal surface of replacement denture.

Case Study 6: Implant case

Mr N. O. – Age 45 years	
Occupation	Doctor
Past medical history	Nil relevant
Social history	Non-smoker
Dental history	Lost the majority of his teeth in adolescence as a result of caries. Has worn upper and lower partial dentures for 20 years.
Complaint	'Looseness of the lower partial denture'. The maxillary partial denture causes no concern.
Clinical assessment	Mucosa appears healthy. Maxillary arch – well-formed ridge (Fig. CS 6.1) Resorbed mandibular ridge (Fig. CS 6.2) Four molar teeth present providing occlusal stops (Fig. CS 6.3).

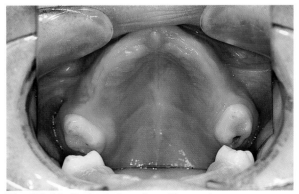

Fig. CS 6.1 Occlusal view of maxillary arch.

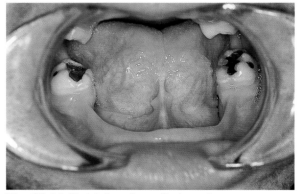

Fig. CS 6.2 Facial view of mandibular arch.

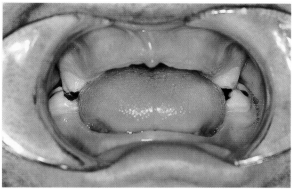

Fig. CS 6.3 The four molar teeth provided centric stops and controlled OVD.

Treatment options

1. Do nothing – maintain present situation
2. New P/P with alternative clasp design
3. Extract the four molars and place C/C
4. Consideration of implant-retained maxillary and mandibular removable prostheses
5. Consideration of maxillary and mandibular implant-retained fixed prostheses.

Discussion

Doing nothing was not considered appropriate by the patient as the looseness of the mandibular denture was becoming socially unacceptable. Replacement of the P/P dentures was an option; however, the likelihood of a predictable improvement was questionable. Extracting the remaining teeth was a possibility in that the retention of a new maxillary denture might be better as the peripheral seal could have been enhanced, but this was not a complaint reported by the patient.

The placement of implants was therefore considered the most preferable treatment option and the procedure was outlined in depth to the patient. An information leaflet was given to the patient for him to peruse and an appointment made with colleagues in oral surgery for further investigation.

It was agreed with the patient to place four implants in the anterior region of the mandible, and this would be followed by construction of an implant-supported removable prosthesis. The patient decided not to have implants placed in the maxillary arch and opted for a new maxillary tissue-supported prosthesis.

Stages

Impressions were made for study casts to enable the fabrication of custom trays for master impressions. These were made and working casts poured. Wax rims were constructed for registration of the jaw relationship. The presence of the posterior teeth significantly aided the measurement of the occlusal vertical dimension, as 'posterior stops' were available. Denture teeth were then set in wax rims (Fig. CS 6.4) and a visit made for the trial dentures to be assessed clinically by both patient and clinician. The trial dentures were considered satisfactory and an acrylic resin replica (Fig. CS 6.5) of the mandibular trial denture was made to act as a guide or template for the surgical placement of the dental implants.

Radiographic examination included taking a dental pantomogram and a lateral jaw view. This enabled the height and width of bone in the anterior region of the mandible to be established. In this particular case no further assessment of the bone architecture was felt necessary, but in

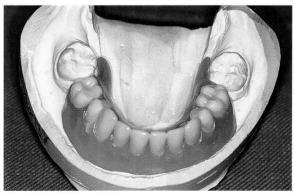

Fig. CS 6.4 Wax trial denture on cast.

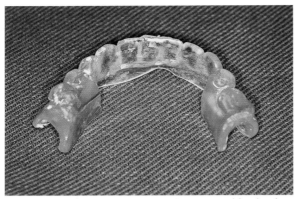

Fig. CS 6.5 Acrylic resin template to guide implant placement.

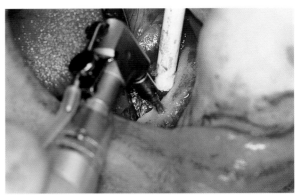

Fig. CS 6.7 An implant is being placed.

some cases bone mapping or scanning radiography is advisable.

The patient was offered intravenous sedation but declined, preferring to have the implants placed under local analgesia alone. The incision made was labial to the anterior mandibular residual ridge (Fig. CS 6.6) and the implants were placed (Fig. CS 6.7). Following insertion of the implants the soft tissues were sutured (Fig. CS 6.8). The patient was instructed not to wear the existing mandibular partial denture for one week, and thereafter the existing denture was lined chairside with a resilient lining material. Three months after implant placement the tissues had healed well (Fig. CS 6.9) and the

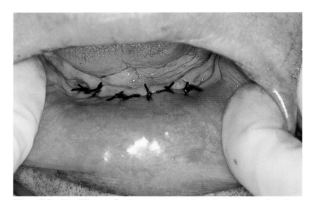

Fig. CS 6.8 The soft tissues were closed over the implant sites.

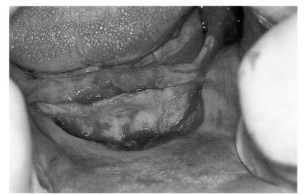

Fig. CS 6.6 The incision was made labial to the crest of the ridge.

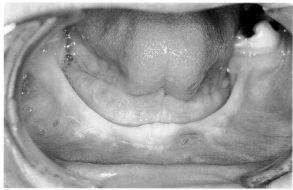

Fig. CS 6.9 Good healing 3 months post-insertion of the implants.

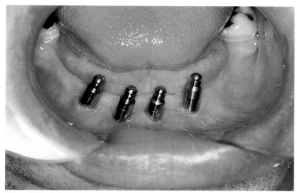

Fig. CS 6.10 Four impression copings in situ.

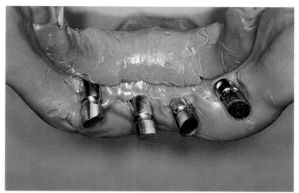

Fig. CS 6.12 Stud and implant body analogues were firmly seated in the definitive impression.

reconstructive phase commenced. This involved second-stage surgery to expose the heads of the dental implants and the placement of healing caps while the existing denture was modified with a chairside soft lining material. Three weeks later the healing caps were unscrewed and impression copings placed (Fig. CS 6.10). Impression material was syringed around the impression copings and the impression tray seated. The impression material was allowed to set and removed for inspection to ensure that adequate detail had been recorded (Fig. CS 6.11). Stud analogues were then placed into the corresponding areas in the impression and implant body analogues attached to the studs (Fig. CS 6.12), which ensured that they

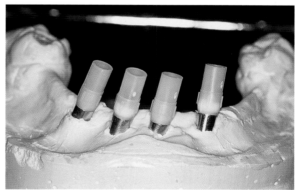

Fig. CS 6.13 Master cast with laboratory analogues inserted over which wax-up sleeves are in place.

were rigidly located in the subsequent cast (Fig. CS 6.13). Shouldered abutments were then chosen and a bar assembly fabricated, and the denture processed.

At the fit stage, the healing caps were removed (Fig. CS 6.14) and shouldered abutments screwed on to the implants (Fig. CS 6.15). The bar assembly was then screwed on to the abutments (Fig. CS 6.16). The clip assembly in the denture is seen in Figure CS 6.17 and in situ in Figure CS 6.18. The patient was instructed in oral hygiene procedures and reviewed three days later. The patient has since been reviewed on a six-monthly basis for maintenance, and is pleased with the final result.

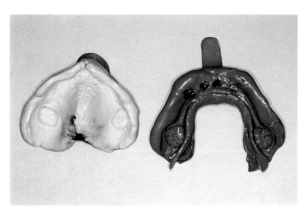

Fig. CS 6.11 The definitive maxillary impressions were recorded.

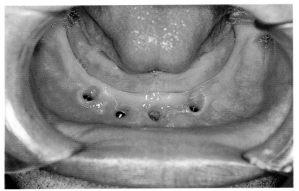

Fig. CS 6.14 The healing caps were removed prior to placement of the shouldered abutments.

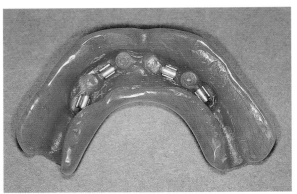

Fig. CS 6.17 View of clip assembly in the impression surface of the mandibular denture.

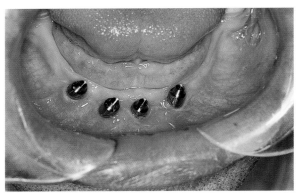

Fig. CS 6.15 Transmucosal shoulder abutments in situ.

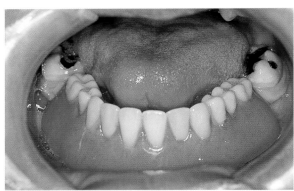

Fig. CS 6.18 The completed mandibular denture was seated in place.

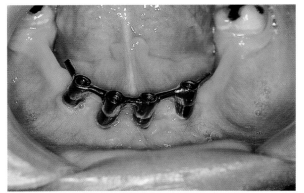

Fig. CS 6.16 The bar assembly was screwed in place.

Case Study 7: Allergy to PMMA

Mrs D. F. – Age 80 years

Occupation	Housewife
Past medical history	Allergies to Savlon, house dust Depression Bruises easily
Medication	Prothiaden, Imipramine, Intal
Dental history	Patient previously had two sets of dentures which, according to her, were 'very old' and worn but comfortable. She experienced problems with the new dentures shortly after they had been inserted. Her mouth became very red and sore (Fig. CS 7.1). The discomfort and soreness began to resolve after the dentures were removed and substituted by the old ones.
Complaint	Recent dentures have caused discomfort and swelling and redness of her mouth. Has had to revert to old dentures.

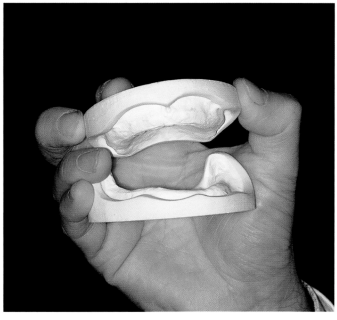

Fig. CS 7.1 Mirror view of palatal tissues showing diffuse erythematous appearance.

Clinical assessment

The maxillary denture-bearing area was erythematous over both the alveolar ridges and the hard palate. Given the clinical picture, denture-induced stomatitis or acrylic allergy were the likeliest possibilities, although the latter was more probable given the history of the complaint. The possibility of an adverse reaction to the new denture material was increased when the dentures were inspected and it was discovered that they were made from polymethylmethacrylate (PMMA) resin, whereas the previous ones were made from vulcanite (Fig. CS 7.2). Special investigations comprised haematology, and culture of swabs taken from the patient's hard palate and maxillary ridges. The haematology results were within normal limits and, surprisingly, swabs taken from the palate and alveolar ridges cultured only a sparse growth of *Candida albicans*; no mycelial elements were identified. Urinalysis was also normal. In the light of these findings acrylic allergy was strongly suspected and the patient was patch tested for the usual battery of tests. This proved that the patient was indeed allergic to PMMA.

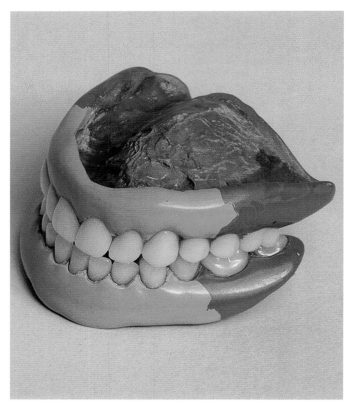

Fig. CS 7.2 The vulcanite dentures with which the patient had been prescribed by a previous practitioner.

Treatment options

1. No active treatment
2. Provision of new dentures using bases not containing PMMA.

Comments

1. No active treatment is a distinct option but would not address the patient's concerns regarding the wear of the previous dentures.

2. Using an alternative denture base material would obviate the need to incorporate PMMA and resolve the discomfort experienced by the patient.

Treatment agreed

Provision of replacement dentures made to usual prosthodontic norms using polycarbonate denture base material (Luxene; Figs CS 7.3, 7.4).

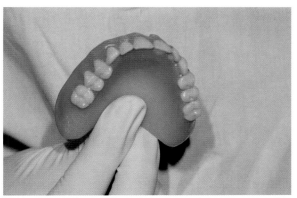

Fig. CS 7.3 The maxillary replacement denture processed in Luxene.

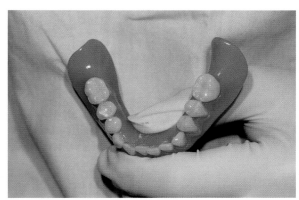

Fig. CS 7.4 The mandibular replacement denture, also processed in Luxene.

Case Study 8: Immediate (transitional) denture

Mrs K. N. – Age 54 years

Occupation	Receptionist
Past medical history	Nil relevant
Social history	Smoker – 30 cigarettes per day
Dental history	Lost the majority of her teeth in middle age as a result of caries/periodontal disease. Has worn a maxillary denture for 10 years, with reasonable success, and has had three sets. The most recent maxillary complete denture was fabricated four years ago.
Complaint	1. Looseness of the mandibular anterior teeth, which also 'bit the lower lip' on eating, causing some discomfort. The looseness was now of such a level that satisfaction in eating was being affected, and more recently the patient reported that speech was also affected.
	2. Looseness of the maxillary denture.
Clinical assessment	Mucosa appeared healthy. Maxillary arch: well formed ridge. Mandibular teeth: the following teeth were present: 34, 33, 32, 31, 41, 42, 43, 44 and 47. Grade III mobility of teeth 32, 31, 41, 42, with probing depths of 7 mm. Grade I mobility of the remaining lower teeth and probing depths less than 4 mm. Generalised bleeding on probing was recorded. A dental pantomogram revealed >90% bone loss associated with the mandibular anterior teeth and approximately 50% with the remainder. A diagnosis of adult periodontitis was made.

Treatment options

1. Do nothing
2. Provision of oral hygiene instruction and periodontal therapy
3. Provision of an immediate mandibular partial denture to replace teeth 32, 31, 41 and 42 following their extraction. Following a period of time for tissue healing, to provide a tooth-supported mandibular cobalt chromium-based partial denture
4. Provision of a resin-retained bridge or a conventional bridge using teeth 33 and 43 as retainers
5. Provision of an implant-retained fixed prosthesis to replace the missing teeth.

Discussion

Doing nothing was not considered appropriate by the patient as the looseness of the teeth was affecting comfort, function and speech. The teeth with the poorest prognosis were considered to be 32, 31, 41 and 42, and the plan therefore concentrated on the fact that these teeth were to be extracted. The management of the periodontal condition was considered essential to help with the long-term prognosis of the remaining mandibular teeth.

The options of fixed and removable solutions to address the missing teeth were discussed with the patient with the aid of photographs and demonstration models. The patient was clear that the having surgery for the placement of dental implants was not an option she wished to follow. The discussion therefore concentrated on the provision of bridgework or dentures. After consideration, the patient felt happiest to proceed with an immediate mandibular partial denture, following the extraction of the mandibular incisor teeth.

Stages

Impressions were made to allow casts to be fabricated, on which custom-made trays were made. The trays were fabricated in light-cured acrylic resin with a wax spacer and finally perforated. Definitive impressions were made and, in the case of the mandibular arch, the large embrasure spaces were blocked out with wax to help prevent the impression material from tearing on removal of the tray. On the resultant casts, registration blocks were fabricated and these were then used to record the occlusal vertical dimension. In addition, appropriate lip support and the mandibular incisal plane were determined. The mould and shade(s) of the replacement teeth were selected and a facebow transfer was performed to allow the casts to be mounted on an articulator (Figs CS 8.1, CS 8.2).

In the mandibular arch, teeth 32, 31, 41 and 42 were ground off at gingival level and the areas of undercut on the cast were blocked out with plaster (Fig. CS 8.3). The mandibular tooth mould was selected in accordance with the

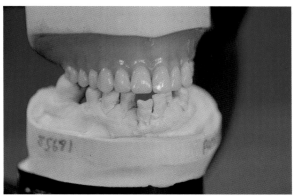

Fig. CS 8.1 After articulation of the cast the maxillary trial denture was set up to the opposing mandibular cast.

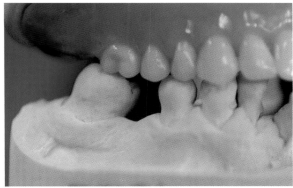

Fig. CS 8.2 Lateral view of the maxillary trial denture opposing the mandibular cast.

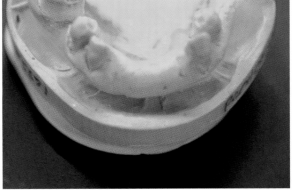

Fig. CS 8.3 The mandibular cast has been prepared by the removal of the incisor teeth plus the blocking out of undesirable undercuts.

dimension of the present teeth. The trial dentures were shown to the patient (Figs CS 8.4, 8.5) and, after approval, the dentures were processed. The patient attended for the extraction of the mandibular incisors, and the maxillary complete denture and immediate mandibular partial denture were inserted after

haemostasis had been achieved. Postoperative instructions, both verbal and written, were given to the patient . The patient was reviewed the next day and adjustments made as required. Tolerance of the prosthesis was good, and following a period of time for tissue healing, a cobalt chromium-based denture was fabricated.

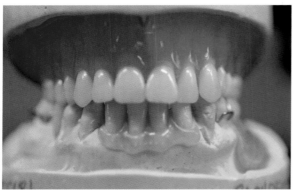

Fig. CS 8.4 Frontal view of trial dentures on articulator.

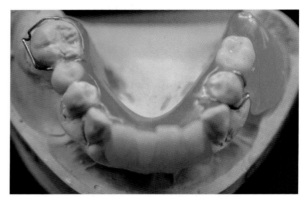

Fig. CS 8.5 Occlusal view of mandibular trial denture.

Index